'Zack George is a true inspi‌‌‌‌ration from humble beginnings to being crowned the UK's fittest man, while transforming the lives of hundreds of others through his CrossFit gym, reminds us that virtually any obstacle can be overcome through a mix of humility, passion, persistence and a supportive community.' – Eric Roza, CEO, CrossFit®

'Zack is the epitome of someone taking control of their life, chasing their dreams, achieving things others only think about. The biggest lesson? Zack isn't special – and I mean that in the nicest possible way. The point is, if he can fulfil his dreams, so can you. His mindset, his dedication, his willingness to graft, have set him apart – and those options are available to us all. Read this book. Improve your life.' – Jake Humphrey, TV presenter and host of *The High Performance Podcast*

START WHERE OTHERS STOP

9 Strategies for Optimising Your Mind

ZACK GEORGE

with David Woolf Morton

SEVEN DIALS

First published in Great Britain in 2021 by Seven Dials
This paperback edition published in 2023 by Seven Dials,
an imprint of The Orion Publishing Group Ltd
Carmelite House, 50 Victoria Embankment
London EC4Y 0DZ

An Hachette UK Company

1 3 5 7 9 10 8 6 4 2

A CIP catalogue record for this book is
available from the British Library.

ISBN (Mass Market Paperback) 978 1 8418 8515 5
ISBN (Audio) 978 1 8418 8505 6
ISBN (eBook) 978 1 8418 8503 2

Typeset by Input Data Services Ltd, Somerset

Printed in Great Britain by Clays Ltd, Elcograf S.p.A.

www.orionbooks.co.uk

CONTENTS

INTRODUCTION

I was born in Leicester in July 1990 and grew up in an area called Evington, about a ten-minute drive from the city centre. It's a normal, quiet suburban town that has retained its village roots and we knew all our neighbours. Everyone would wish each other good morning and it was a comfortable place to bring up a family. I've always lived in Leicestershire and I still do. But growing up as a kid, I was *very* different to how I am today – I certainly didn't look anything like how I do on the cover of this book! Instead, I was dangerously overweight, lazy and almost completely inactive.

Now, as I write this, I am the UK's fittest man – something I've achieved through years of training as a professional athlete in the sport of CrossFit. If you're unfamiliar with CrossFit, it's one of the most demanding and gruelling sports to train for and compete in, combining almost every discipline of fitness you can think of. You've got to be able to run and swim long distances but strong enough to lift heavy barbells above your head; you need to have the muscular power to push a sled or throw a sandbag, yet also be highly skilled in gymnastic movements like handstands. In competitions, it's not uncommon to be challenged on all those abilities and more in a single workout. It makes sense, then, that the man and woman crowned champions at our marquee event, the CrossFit Games, are dubbed 'the fittest on earth'.

But almost nobody who knew me as a young child would have picked me out to be a professional athlete. I wouldn't have guessed it for myself either, to be honest, yet here we are! As I've mentioned, I was an overweight and lazy kid, partly because I loved junk food more than anything, and it's not hard to imagine how my life might well have turned out differently. I could now, so easily, be unhealthy, unfit and far too heavy, completely uncomfortable with my state of mind and working a job I'd fallen into and had zero passion for.

When I tell people about my background, they always ask me, 'How did you do it? How did you go from a chubby kid scoffing sweets to the fittest man in the UK?' The truth is that it hasn't been a straightforward transformation. Over the years, I have tried to become a professional rugby player, I've worked as a personal trainer at a run-of-the-mill health club, I've had my own group workout business, opened two gyms and even had to close one before it bankrupted me. I've tasted failure of every sort in the process but I've savoured every success, too.

2

Perhaps the greatest outcome of all of these ups and downs, however, has been that they have forged in me a certain mindset, one that I rely upon in every single part of my life. I call it 'Start Where Others Stop'. It's a mantra I repeat to myself when I'm training in the gym and gasping for air, it's a way of thinking that I apply to my business life to push myself to try new things and it is a declaration that I will always go the extra mile for my loved ones.

But the Start Where Others Stop mindset is not some kind of secret door to which only I have the key. It is a mentality that can be learned and that you can develop yourself and apply to your own life, whatever the dream you have in mind or the challenges you might face. That is why I wanted to write this book, to share with you how to formulate that mindset and give you the tools to set goals, overcome hurdles and achieve anything.

In this book, I have split the Start Where Others Stop mindset up into nine strategies, which stack up on top of each other to construct this resilient mentality. I'm going to share with you the experiences, events and people who have shaped me as a person and forged my approach to provide some context as we build your way of thinking and, along the way, I'm going to give you the exercises and activities that have helped me, so that you too can better understand your development. Then, at the end of each of the nine chapters, you'll find your Start Where Others Stop (SWOS) programme, which will let you evaluate where you are and build an unbreakable mindset brick by brick, from establishing your goals to learning from failure and achieving your dreams. At the back of the book, you'll find pages where you can fill in these exercises as you go along so you have a record of where you are and how far you've come.

Deep down, we all have dreams that we would love to reach for and make real. It may be a huge goal, like transforming your body when you've never really done any exercise before, or it could be completing a marathon having only ever run for the bus. Maybe you're targeting a big promotion at work or saving money to move your family into a new home. Perhaps your wishes are smaller, like learning the guitar, or much broader, such as being a better friend, parent or partner. It could be that you simply want to be a more positive sort of person.

It doesn't matter what your personal goals are. All goals are equal. If it's important to you, if it's something that has always been in the back of your mind and you wish it could become real, it counts. You can work towards it and, with the mentality we are going to build together, you can achieve anything. Picking up this book is the beginning. Now all you need to do is get a start. This is how I got mine.

PART I
SET GOALS

CHAPTER ONE

ANYONE CAN MAKE A START

There are moments you never forget, even though they happened when you were just a kid. I remember my mum taking me to our local supermarket one day and I'd never seen it so busy. The car park was rammed and I sat in the back seat staring out the window as Mum went round and round looking for a space. When finally one became free, she reversed in and I suddenly noticed how far from the shop we were. I know they say that when you're little everything seems huge but to me, that distance looked like miles.

I immediately started whingeing. Even though I was only seven years old, I was already overweight and I hated walking anywhere, so the distance from the car to the supermarket door immediately set me off. I begged Mum to wait a bit to see if a closer parking space opened up and in a desperate attempt to avoid the exercise, I told her I wouldn't get out of the car until it did. She looked at me in the rearview mirror and told me that I would be OK, that it wasn't that far and that we'd do it together. 'You can do it, Zack,' she said. Eventually, we got out and walked to the shop.

By the time I was eight, I was still overweight but, even though I had remained lazy, I had developed a love for sports, which would at least get me moving around at school with my friends. But even though I liked playing football and tennis, because of my weight I would get tired and pack it in after 20 minutes. I remember my parents trying everything they could to get me to go out on a walk with the family at the weekend and I would kick up a massive fuss. While I could just about motivate myself to play a bit of football at lunchtime, I had zero interest in any physical activity they tried to get me into.

Trying to understand what led me to be so averse to exercising, I think it all stemmed from my mum wanting to have a huge family. Mum wanted seven or eight kids! She had my sister, Martine, in 1983 and then there was a seven-year gap before I came along. During that time, Mum had five or six miscarriages, which is about one a year, give or take. But she wanted more children, so they just kept trying. When she was pregnant with me, she pretty much rested the entire time because she was so worried about losing me.

When I came along, Mum was just so happy and grateful to have another kid that she smothered me with love and affection. I could do nothing wrong. If I wanted sweets or chocolate, she would give them to me. My dad would always say, 'You've got to stop feeding him that!' but she would do it anyway because it made me happy, which made her happy. However, this did mean that there were a lot of arguments between Mum and Dad about my diet and my weight.

Every day after school, I would eat a giant bag of Haribo and I practically inhaled chocolate. Mum would take me to KFC and I'd order a family bargain bucket to take home, pick off all the skin and leave the chicken. I would sit on the sofa with a big grin on my face, eating only the 'bad' bit and chucking the protein – the part that's even vaguely good for you – in the bin. By the time I was ten, when we went to McDonald's I'd order a supersized McChicken meal with a milkshake and twenty nuggets. I finished it all no problem.

On Friday evenings, Dad would always go out to play cards, so Mum and I had 'snack night'. It would always be an insane amount of food and it was amazing. We'd get a tray, put five or six chocolate bars on it, loads of packs of crisps and tons of sweets, then we'd go up to my room together and tuck in. It sounds awful now but I used to love Friday nights with Mum – they are really happy memories. We could only do that because Dad was out of the house and didn't know what we were doing.

Mum loved it too because she was spending time with me and, back then, she was also really into sweets and chocolate. She's definitely who I get my sweet tooth from! My dad and my sister have never been that bothered and just have a few sweets here and there. Whereas me and Mum, well, if we've got five chocolate bars in front of us we can't leave a single one of them!

Whenever Mum bought sweets for my sister and me there would be arguments. I'd eat all mine within two minutes and Martine would have pretty much all of hers left, saving them for later in the day. Then I'd go and eat hers and we'd have a row about it. I just couldn't help myself. So Mum would get another chocolate bar out of the cupboard to keep the peace. She was so soft and loving that we could get away with anything.

If you're wondering why I'm telling you this, it's because understanding where I come from and how I was raised has been such an important step for me in making a change to my life. When we're thinking about taking our first step, we have to understand where we come from before we start moving towards that new goal. It could be the context and environment you were brought up in, or maybe just how things have been going at work for the last few months. All our experiences mould our outlook and attitudes, so if you can try to consider what has brought you to where you are, you can start out in the right direction. We'll delve further into this at the end of the chapter when we begin building your Start Where Others Stop programme.

BE POSITIVE

Proper goal setting starts with the language you use to describe your goals, even if that is just talking to yourself at this stage. Positive statements are much more likely to motivate you than negative ones, so always frame your goals with a positive statement. Rather than telling yourself, 'I'm not going to be as lazy,' instead think of it as 'I will be a more active person.' Or in place of, 'I want to eat less junk food,' say 'I am going to eat a balanced diet.'

A study published in the *Social Cognitive and Affective Neuroscience* journal found that having a positive outlook actually changes neural mechanisms and makes behaviour change more likely. Start thinking like this from the very beginning and you're setting yourself up for success already.

My parents came from nothing. My dad moved over from Guyana at the age of 11. His childhood in South America was a very different way of life compared to what we've all become used to now, in this country. They didn't have TV, sure, but they also had to catch their own food. It was very basic. His dad died quite early on too, in a diving accident at sea, so he had a pretty harsh start.

Dad's mum moved over to Leicester in the early 1960s but didn't have enough money to bring the kids with her to begin with, so dad, his two brothers and his little sister stayed with family friends back in Guyana while his mum, my grandmother, saved up as much money as she could. After a year, she could only afford to bring one of them over, so their sister was sent for first. My dad has since told me that when their father was alive he was very strict, so all the kids adored their mum. Dad has given me the impression it was really tough on them when she moved away. Each year, another one of them made the trip and it went on like that, year after year, with my grandmother working hard and saving almost everything she had to bring her children back together here in England.

When Dad finally arrived in 1965, the UK was still very segregated. Back then, if you were Black you had to deal with a lot of racial abuse and it was hardcore. I can't count the number of stories he's told me of fights he had just because a group of white lads saw him and it all kicked off and it built a hardness and toughness into him. How could it not? Although it was a different time, recent events around the world that have reignited protests and demands for racial equality suggest that things aren't entirely different now. We've had our own share of issues in the CrossFit community, even.

Dad met my mum at school in 1967, so they've known each other since they were only 13 years old and now they're 66 and still together, which is pretty rare. For parents to be together full stop is good going these days! It wasn't easy though – when they were dating properly as young teenagers in the late sixties and they started going to clubs and dances a Black man being out with a white woman caused a lot of problems.

The attitude in Britain in the sixties was that if you were Black, you dated a Black person; if you were white, you dated a white person. So they had to keep their relationship hidden for six or seven years, as it simply wasn't the accepted or 'normal' thing to do. Both sets of parents weren't happy that their child was dating someone of another colour and that went on for a while. As it happens, though, in the end my nan, my mum's mum, split up with Grandad and started dating a Black person – it's funny how things turn out.

My parents had it hard growing up, as not only did they have to deal with the racial abuse they received as an interracial couple in the sixties and seventies but they also had very little money. They've always been a huge inspiration to me in this regard, as they never had anything handed to them. Everything was earned. Together they built a textiles business from scratch, starting off in the Leicester markets. Bill and Jean Adderley, who started Dunelm, had a little stall next to them! The now retail giant Next had a shop on the corner and was stocked with just a few basic T-shirts. They all started in the same place, in Leicester markets, and then made their way up from there.

The house my parents lived in, the house we grew up in,

they managed to buy when they were 21 and it was massive, with six bedrooms, a snooker table and a jacuzzi. They worked their fingers to the bone for every penny of that house.

Running a business as a Black person back then, however, you were always at a disadvantage. If my dad had a product that looked amazing but a white competitor was offering something that was half as good, a buyer would go with the white person the majority of the time just because they were white. To get anywhere, to be as successful as he was, Dad had to be extremely resilient and very forceful and he quickly became known as a hard nut. He had to try and be smarter than everyone else. He had to be ruthless. He had to be tough.

Obviously, that bled into our home life. If you're in business for a couple of decades, having to graft harder than other people because of your skin colour, it's going to impact your whole way of thinking and acting. As a result, he was strict – very strict at times – and he often made us do things that we didn't want to do. I remember he would sit us down and have us recite the times tables and we couldn't leave until we'd got it right. Even when we went on holiday we had to do it.

Martine had it worse than I did, though. Because she's seven years older, he was extremely strict for the vast majority of her childhood, so much so she moved out of home when she was 16 and lived in a hostel for about a year or two. I was nine and I remember her moving out but I didn't know why or what was happening. Dad was just quite regimented with everything back then and it was exhausting. Luckily for me, when he retired aged 40, he started to slowly chill out bit by bit. He had to try to calm down a bit for us and my mum. Mum's always been there for us. Her sole purpose was and still is to give us the best life she could.

Retired or not though, Dad was still pretty straight-down-the-line and the sort of stuff I ate and how overweight I was became a regular flashpoint at home. There were lots of arguments where Dad would say 'Stop feeding him that! Stop giving him sweets!' Of course he was right but he was going about it the wrong way. I remember messing around and wrestling with him on the lounge floor. For some reason I used to have a phobia about being on my back. I hated it. So Dad would get me on my back then hold me there while I was kicking and screaming, saying 'get over it!' It sounds bad but he was a loving father and just wanted us to face our fears so we could be in control of our lives.

I didn't understand why he was doing it at the time but I can see now that my dad never wanted our potential to be limited by being afraid. He was teaching me that putting yourself in a difficult position is the only way to overcome your anxieties or worries. Those first few times he got me on my back I panicked but he talked to me and encouraged me to calm down, and before long I didn't have a problem with it any more.

Unconventional as his method was, it taught me that if you're scared of something or you have a weakness you'd like to work on, the best place to start is to knowingly put yourself in that position, making sure you remain calm and collected with your thoughts. If you're scared of speaking in public and want to become better at giving presentations or even simply talking more in meetings, trading that panic for a clearer mind will give you the perspective you need to understand where to begin improving. Chances are, you'll realise there is much less to worry about than you thought.

That's not to say it's easy, though. As you might imagine, I was very self-conscious about my body and I'd never have my top off in public. On the days we had swimming at school, I would say to my mum that I wasn't feeling too good and she would let me stay at home. I thought I was being really smart but of course my mum knew what I was doing.

I was confident enough in myself around my family. My sister and I would draw a six-pack on to my big belly and I'd run around pretending I was ripped. I'd take the piss out of myself and do a dance where I'd wobble my belly. The whole family would be cracking up. But having my body on show in front of other people was a totally different thing altogether. I remember sitting in the lounge one day with my top off and seeing a family friend's car suddenly pull in. Nobody had told me they were coming and I started to run upstairs to put a T-shirt on but Dad caught hold of me on the way out the door and said: 'You shouldn't be afraid of your body – just sit here!' I started crying and there was a bit of an argument as Mum wanted me to go and get a top on if that would make me happy. I ended up going upstairs and putting something on before our guests came in but that's how little confidence I had in myself physically at the time.

At school, I was quite lucky – I didn't really get picked on because I was so friendly and I got on well with everyone. There were lots of groups at school but I was always the one who floated around and was 'in' with everyone, I was a character. I had my main group of friends but then I'd still hang out with other people as well. When I was playing sport, the other teams would often call me fat and that sort of thing but it never got to me too much. Despite not being that sure of myself, other people's comments didn't really affect me and by the age of ten I was starting to really enjoy rugby – I could just bulldoze the other team over!

But even though I got on with my friends at school, I was very family focused, so most of the time I was at home I'd be with my mum. There were a few kids on the street that I mucked around with and we'd go to the shops and get sweets sometimes, though I wasn't one of these kids that was out of the house much. My mum encouraged me to do stuff with other people but as soon as I got home, I just wanted to chill. I felt more comfortable there and I was so close to my mum; after the trouble she went through having me, she wanted to spend as much time with me as possible, too. We didn't really do much and we didn't need to. All I wanted was to go home and be with mum, to sit together, watch TV and have some food.

PUT PEN TO PAPER

There is a part of the human brain that is crucial to goal setting and it regulates our actions as we move towards that goal. The reticular activating system (RAS) is a cluster of cells at the base of the brain which is responsible for handling all the information related to things that are demanding our attention at the moment. It is why you tend to notice something more often when you're thinking about it, such as seeing a certain model of car everywhere when you are considering buying the same model. They were there all along, of course, but the RAS is triggering you to be more aware of them.

Conveniently, the RAS can be co-opted while setting goals and increase the likelihood of success from the very first stage. According to research by the department of psychology at Emory University in Atlanta, USA, all you have to do is put pen to paper. Write down three objectives on a piece of paper and place it somewhere where you will see it regularly – maybe on the fridge or the back of your front door. Try to limit yourself to three, as having too long a list will limit how often you stop to read them. Seeing your objectives regularly allows that part of your brain to make you more aware of your aims. It is a simple method to ensure on a neurological level you are motivated to go for it and make a start.

We ended up moving to a new house when I was 12 and it was a massive thing for me. My sister and I absolutely loved the house we grew up in and we cried our eyes out as we were leaving but the house was just too big. We moved to Tur Langton, which is still Leicestershire, but outside of Leicester. It's a lovely village surrounded by countryside but at the time I didn't want to move and I couldn't see the point. I distinctly remember my mum saying that there was a McDonald's only two minutes' drive away and, funnily enough, I was more into it then!

By the time I was 13, rugby had become my complete focus, as I struggled with the academic side of school but found my size really helped me on the rugby field. I was surprisingly fast, even though I was overweight for my age, and I was the dominant player in my team. My nickname was 'the Washing Machine' because I was solid and immovable! Playing well and smashing people in matches was who I was at that time. I started to get a few knee issues, though, and my feet were getting flatter and flatter as a result of carrying more and more weight as I grew. I didn't recognise it but Dad did. He was thinking about what would happen if I got too big, about whether I'd get picked on when I went to secondary school.

He knew I was gifted at sport and wanted me to have the physical ability to play to a higher level.

Recently I found out that my dad had tried a handful of times to find a way to help me lose some weight over the course of two to three years before secondary school. Apparently, he would chat to me about eating more healthily and cutting down on the junk food but I'd just ignore him. To be honest, I don't remember.

What is really vivid in my mind, though, is the event that got me started on the path to where I am today. It wasn't an ultimatum from Dad, or a case of me having a moment of clarity about where I wanted my life to go. It was only the first step and a little one at that. It was a PlayStation 2.

A new games console coming out is a massive thing when you're 13. The PlayStation 2 was just mind-blowing to me; some of the other kids at school were getting them and I was desperate for one. I knew my dad wouldn't just buy it for me – he'd make me earn it in some way. He always wanted to make us understand the real value of things and now I understand the importance of that, of how he came from nothing and built an amazing life for his family brick by brick.

As a 13-year-old boy, though, I just wanted it and because he had tried so many different things to get me to lose weight without any success, he gave bribery a shot – the PS2 was the carrot at the end of the stick. He sat me down and said, 'Let's make a deal. I'm going to give you three weeks and if you lose some weight, I'll get you the PlayStation.' We agreed that he

ANYONE CAN MAKE A START

would weigh and measure me on that third weekend and if I'd managed to shift some weight, we would go straight to the shops together and buy one.

He told me all I had to do was cut down on what I was eating and I was so excited at the prospect of a new games console that I bought in completely. Instead of going to McDonald's four or five times a week, I went once or twice a week. I didn't have chocolate so often and stopped eating a bag of Haribo after school every day (though I still did it some days). I didn't feel like I was eating that much less but I was cutting out a huge chunk of the junk food and, even though I wasn't doing any extra exercise, that simple reduction in crap calories meant the weight started falling off. It came off *really* easily. I could see my tummy shrinking a bit and I started to feel better about myself. When it came to the last weekend of the challenge, we got the tape measure and scales out. I'll never forget looking down at the tape.

Whenever we did anything vaguely good at home or at school, Mum would always make a massive fuss about it and shower us in praise. Not Dad, though. All you'd get out of him was an occasional nod, or sometimes a 'you did fine', maybe even a 'good job'. But when he passed the tape around my belly and checked the measurement, he just looked at me and beamed. He was so happy, he jumped up and hugged me and told me how proud of me he was. Then, exactly as he'd promised, he grabbed our coats and drove me straight to Toys-R-Us.

PUSH YOURSELF A LITTLE FURTHER

When you are first getting to grips with goal setting, it is helpful to start with something you feel as though you can realistically achieve, then push yourself by going one step further.

Research at Yale University discovered that 'stability' – predictable and easy tasks – switches off the parts of your brain responsible for adaptation, whereas 'instability' – the less predictable and hard – fires up your ability to improve and learn.

At work, for example, if you think hitting your deadlines is attainable, challenge yourself by setting yourself false deadlines so that you always have time to review and improve your work before the real deadline comes along. Going slightly out of your comfort zone is the shortcut to sustainable personal development.

I loved that PlayStation. Though it sounds counterintuitive to be sitting down playing video games having just lost weight, it represented something bigger. It was the first time that I felt a sense of real achievement. It felt amazing. We set a goal, gave it a realistic time frame and then worked to achieve it. Sure, I was still overweight, but I had realised that by starting towards a goal and then sticking to it, I was capable of more than I thought and, even though it had only been three weeks, I had built the first foundations of real resilience. Each time I didn't give in to the cravings for a chocolate bar or the desire to beg Mum to take me to McDonalds, it further proved to me the power of a bit of mental fortitude.

I understand now how the weeks of eating a little bit better, my dad's pride when he passed the tape around my tummy and then plugging in that PlayStaion 2 for the first time changed my perspective of what I was capable of achieving. It sowed the seed that personal growth was possible if you wanted it and that finding the motivation to start was the key.

Every parent sets goals for their children and offers a reward of some sort − whether that's to brush their teeth, tidy their room or try harder at school. It's just that my formative experience of losing that bit of weight when I was so unhealthy was more on the extreme end of the scale. Ultimately, it comes down to my dad having to grow up so fast and not having the luxury of both parents looking after him, or enough money to get by. He was left behind in Guyana and then moved to a completely different country when he was 11 years old, to an area where a person with his skin colour wasn't really wanted. His mental resilience was forged by that experience and, in turn, I was being shaped by that context. So much of what he did was to instil in us that same

ANYONE CAN MAKE A START

If we're all honest with ourselves, the first obstacle is always getting started. We can become paralysed by the endgame, by the myriad stairs we will have to get up as we climb towards our goals. The concept of tripping or falling along the way can stop us from ever taking that first step at all. So, too often, we don't bother even starting.

No matter the magnitude of your goal, your time frame or how you will measure success, *just get started*. Ignore the voice in your head telling you that it would be easier not to take that first step. Once you've made the little jump from thinking about doing something to actually doing it, you can move onto establishing the smaller stages that will help you build towards your bigger ambition.

Anyone can make a start. The sooner you get cracking on achieving your goals – be they huge dreams or your daily to-do list – the easier it becomes to get started next time and soon you will be the sort of person who is always busy getting better.

YOUR SWOS PROGRAMME

Welcome to your Start Where Others Stop programme. As we move through this book, we're going to be building upon how you approach goals, tackle challenges and achieve your aims. Your version of the SWOS mindset is entirely personal to you, so the more thought you give to each exercise and the harder you try to relate each question to yourself, the better your unique programme will become. At the back of the book there's a section where you can fill in the exercises you'll find on the SWOS Programme pages at the end of each chapter. It's important to keep your answers together somewhere safe, as we're going to be referring back to previous parts of the plan as we move on. If you'd prefer not to write in the book itself, a notebook is perfect and you can also make notes on your phone, as and when things occur to you. I do that all the time.

First of all, we're going to consider where we come from and where we'd like to get to. We are all shaped by our environments, be that the home you grew up in, where you work, or the people you spend your free time with.

Building your understanding of where you come from is an important first stage of goal setting as it helps you key into why those goals are important to you on a deeper and more motivating level.

When you have a goal in mind, ask yourself the following questions. As mentioned, the process of writing can have a hugely positive effect, so do try and note down your answers on page 227 or somewhere else:

1) WHO ARE YOU?

What are the three defining characteristics of your personality? They can be positive or negative. Who is responsible for the instilling of those traits? Are there any events that have been responsible? Don't forget that some might be your doing.

2) WHERE WOULD YOU LIKE TO GO?

Now reconsider your goal having thought about what has shaped you as a person. Is the destination the right one? Do you need to alter it slightly to take into account your attitudes and experiences?

3) WHAT WILL GET YOU THERE?

Finally, try to identify the primary positive action that will start you on the road to progress. What change will make the largest impact? This is your starting point and in the next chapter we will establish the smaller steps you need to take to make things happen.

CHAPTER TWO

TAKE SMALL STEPS TO ACHIEVE BIG DREAMS

The person I had become by the time I was a young adult couldn't have been more different to that lad sat happily playing on the PlayStation. But looking back now, I realise that I had already started to transform mentally and physically. Mum poured me full of love and Dad planted that seed of belief that you can do anything, that if you just start, then you're already on your way to a better version of yourself, regardless of your target.

As I've said, though, it certainly wasn't a straight line from chubby kid to the fittest man in the UK. You need to put in place smaller steps that keep you moving towards your goal so you make the incremental gains that add up to a transformation of any type and size.

Think of it like running five kilometres. If your aim is to finish in 30 minutes, simply starting your stopwatch then setting off at top speed and hoping you'll manage it doesn't make sense. If you've ever gone out too fast on a run then you know very well that you will end up bent over, sucking in oxygen and then trudging slowly onwards with your hands on your head. But if you split that five kilometres into one-kilometre segments, then you know that you just need to finish each section in six minutes in order to hit your target total time, so you go at the right pace from the start and tick off each kilometre as it passes.

The only way to make it to your finish line is to take one step at a time. Sometimes you'll be able to put your head down and go faster; often you'll have to go slowly but surely, taking care where you put your feet. When you do have to slow down, you know there is only a little further before you can tick off another section of your race and start picking up the pace again. Done right, it means you can finish strong, rather than limping over the line.

Breaking up a goal into smaller, more manageable micro-goals is the most rewarding way to get to where you want to be. Everything can be divided into incremental improvements towards a grander purpose. In the gym, for example, your goal might be to get really strong. But if you just go and load all the plates you can find onto a barbell and try to lift it, you won't be able to and you won't build any strength at all.

Setting yourself a target for the month of adding ten kilograms to your bench press, then dividing the month into four weeks and every gym session into even smaller goals that are easier to tick off – like not missing any of your planned training days or being able to bench press your previous personal best for an extra repetition at the end of each week – is infinitely easier to grasp. At the end of that month, you might well surprise yourself by being adding 15kg to your record. Which is something worth celebrating before setting your next target and working out what steps you need to take in order to keep improving.

If you were only able to manage an extra five kilograms, that is the moment that your mentality can take a bit of the load. You haven't missed your goal. Your aim was to get really strong and you have undeniably increased your strength. That five-kilogram plate is empirical proof that you have improved and moved closer to your bigger dream. Now all you have to do is work out what steps you can take to get to that ten kilogram increase and beyond.

You can apply this to every area of your life. If your dream is to make a drastic career change that will transform your way of life, or just finally get round to decorating your home how you've always wanted it, seeing each step and making them one by one will keep you moving in the right direction.

SET REALLY MICRO-GOALS

We all tend to believe that the better version of ourselves is attainable. It's human nature. But we also tend to think that either huge changes or fast fixes will result in achieving our goals. Yet it is daily choices or micro-goals that have a positive neurobiological impact on our brain.

Scientists at Harvard and the University of Southern California found that even small 'tokens', such as crossing things off a list, motivated people to keep working towards the bigger goal. Micro-goals can rewire your brain, flooding it with dopamine – the 'feel-good' hormone – each and every time you tick one off. Even simple, daily tasks such as doing the washing-up or putting the bins out provide you with that buzz.

Rather than focusing on your end goal, consider what small tasks you can complete tomorrow that will contribute to meeting your objectives, no matter how little they are. *Harvard Business Review* researchers found that smaller wins actually increase a person's happiness and the more frequently they experience that sense of progress, the more chance they have of continuing to be successful in their larger goals.

Let's start by listing three micro-goals you can get done today. They should be simple things, like finishing this chapter, clearing your inbox or going for a walk. Write them down and then make a point of stopping for a moment to cross them off one by one as you finish them. Savour that buzz. Each one on its own isn't hard to achieve but the sense of achievement you feel when they are all ticked off at the end of the day is the power of taking small steps in action.

In the time between me and Dad hitting that first goal and when I moved up into the next school year, I continued slowly losing weight. By the time I was 14, I was pretty much a regular kid. I was a bit tubby and was known for drinking Fanta all the time and having a sweet tooth but I was nowhere near as fat as I was before. I still loved rugby and now that I wasn't as heavy, I could play harder for longer, run faster and further. It was a good feeling.

That year, Dad took the whole family to a three-day seminar in Birmingham being given by Tony Robbins, an American self-help author and speaker whose books and events were immensely popular at the time. I remember moaning about having to go and asking Dad why I couldn't just hang out with my friends instead. It wasn't the sort of thing that appeals when you're a 14-year-old lad. But as much as I hate to admit it, the trip turned out to be a life-changing few days. We spoke a lot about mental strength and self-empowerment, of course, but there was also loads of stuff about your nutrition and your health and how that can help you to be successful in your everyday life. I started taking notice.

If you've ever seen anything about those seminars online, you'll know that they gear you up over the three days for this huge event at the end where you literally walk over hot coals. We listened to the talks, finding out all this information about what you can achieve if you put your mind to it and how, if you want to be successful in life, your health and mindset is vitally important. We got to the end of each long day exhausted but thrilled, filled with the feeling that you can conquer anything. It was a full-on environment.

So, when it came to the last day, we lined up with the other hundreds of people at the seminar ready to walk down this pathway of hot coals. Looking back now, obviously it's just a gimmick. The staff make it out like you're walking across lava but it probably wasn't that hot at all. As a kid though, it made a huge impression on me. Everyone was running over the coals and there were people cheering at the other end. Before I knew it, it was our turn and we walked across it, all of us, as a family.

It signified a massive mental shift for us. Whether it was the seminar itself or simply the experience of going through that process of self-evaluation together, we immediately shifted into a different gear and when we got home we threw out all the Christmas chocolates the next day. I had taken loads of sweets on the trip with me but they all went in the bin. We went vegetarian and Dad started researching health and nutrition and went on a massive fitness kick. The entire family was energised; we were vegetarian for six or seven years and then pescatarian after that.

For me, the boost in self-confidence was perfectly timed. I was suddenly fired up to get healthy for myself. No bribes or deals or PlayStations – this time it was for *me*. I decided I wanted to get fit and excel at sport and I wanted to set myself up to have a good career in anything I chose to pursue. It was a powerful time for me as a young person. I started to be known locally as the sporty kid and, as I lost weight and got leaner, I became the fastest, strongest and fittest, both in my school and in our corner of Leicestershire. The self-belief I had in myself and the confidence that I could do something if I set my mind to it evolved by the day. It was addictive, almost.

It was around that point, that I started to become good at rugby, so I made it my goal to reach the top in the sport and my dream then was to be a professional rugby player. Students at Ratcliffe College, which I attended, also played hockey and cricket but rugby was the main event and the whole school turned out to watch the big games. When we were in the lower years at the school, we would watch the first XV play and look at the year 13 lads, the 18 year olds, and just think they were gods. They were grown men to us. Occasionally, if somebody was good enough, the coaches would pick a player from year 11 to play in the first XV when they were only 15–16 years old. It was rare, but it was possible. I decided I would do everything I could to be one of those picked a year early.

The coming season, I got selected for the first XV. It was only me and a guy called Daniel Sleeth who were deemed good enough to play up a year and we thought we were kings. Everyone else our age seemed to agree with us; it seemed like such a big deal to get selected to represent the school so young.

Disappointingly though, I didn't enjoy playing for the first XV at all. That whole year, I got absolutely hammered by guys three years older than me, in training and especially during matches against other schools. I was playing fully grown men and, even though I was now fit and strong, I was getting dominated when I had become so used to being top dog. Every game was hard and my mum didn't like it because she could see how much bigger the older people I was playing against were. It hurt and I didn't look forward to the games. I hated it, really, and would be wracked with nerves on a Saturday morning before the matches. I was young for my year, so I was only just 15 when I started in the team. I was probably one of the youngest to ever do it, which, although quite an achievement, made it hard for me to compete physically.

I could have stopped playing for the first XV, gone back to being a force in my own year's team and running rampant against boys my age but I stuck it out. I wasn't aware of it, but the mindset that had been given life by my dad and that we, as a family, had committed to earlier that year meant that giving up was never an option. I turned up to every practice and played every game. At the start of the season, I didn't think I would make it to the end and I couldn't imagine getting through it. Yet by going to the first training session and then the next and the one after that, by turning up to the matches week in and week out, I was taking the smaller steps to completing a whole season for the first XV when I was only 15 years old.

The self-confidence that experience built was a gamechanger for me. I won awards that year at the end of the season and I started playing representative rugby for Leicestershire. I was improving and hitting the micro-goals I was setting myself along the way, taking the steps towards playing professionally.

I started getting scouted by the Tigers Academy. When I was growing up, Leicester Tigers were one of the best professional teams in the whole country and were always in contention to win the premiership, so when their junior section started to get interested in me joining with a view to moving up through the age grades and perhaps even being awarded a professional contract, it proved I was definitely moving in the right direction.

It was a step-up physically but by the time I was 17 that was no longer an issue, as I'd more than caught up with my strength and fitness, which was starting to really take off. I was now known as the 'fitness kid' around Leicester. The training at the Tigers Academy was more serious − for example, they monitored our weight training and gave us some great advice on nutrition for proper performance − and further boosted my development as an athlete.

Most influential, though, was the mindset of everyone there, from the players to the coaches, even the parents.

When you're playing rugby at school, it's part of your normal week and almost everyone plays, whether they are genuinely talented or just decent enough to make the top teams, so you have a laugh during training and even muck around during matches when you're winning. But the Tigers were different. Everyone was there for one reason and that was to get better. The coaches weren't teachers who also ran a team or two around their classes, they considered it their job to identify and develop the next generation of professionals for the Leicester Tigers. We took our training sessions seriously and treated each one as a chance to improve, both on and off the field. It was a huge opportunity for me and such a positive step towards my bigger goal. I was determined to go at it at full speed.

DECIDE HOW IMPORTANT IT IS

When you have set a goal, work out how important it is for you to achieve it. Simply by thinking about how much you want to make those things happen relative to the other priorities in your life makes you much more likely to take positive steps in your day-to-day life.

In fact, a mathematician at the University of Pittsburgh researching decision making found that 'zooming out' in this way is a vital tool in establishing your priorities within your overall goal. It will also help you see the bigger picture in the small moments. If spending time with your family is your goal, realising how important that is compared to, say, working late in the office, will make leaving on time an easier thing to do. Take a moment now to think about how important your goal is to you in comparison to other areas of your life.

Unfortunately though, my body couldn't keep pace with my ambition to play professional rugby. While I was training with the Tigers Academy, I ran head first into an opponent I simply couldn't out-muscle: injury. You get little niggles when you're playing for your school, you pull a small muscle or dislocate a finger or two. Certainly nothing crazy and it never stops you for long. But when I was 17, I started to suffer from collapsed arches, the result of all those years I'd been so heavy and the flat-footed running style Dad had noticed back when I was still called 'the Washing Machine'.

Because my feet were collapsing, I started to sprain my ankles all the time. If I played five games, I probably had to come off the field in four of them with a rolled ankle. I was angry and frustrated whenever it happened. It didn't seem fair that I was just entering such an important phase of my rugby, seriously thinking about it as a career, only to get injured all the time. I went to see a few different physios and foot specialists, and it was quickly established that my flat feet were causing not just problems with my ankles but knee and hip issues, too.

I kept playing, though, as I had stuck it out when it was tough facing opponents three years older than me at school, and was determined that I would make it through with the Tigers. When I was 18, I spent almost the entire season getting injured, doing weeks of rehab and then coming back, only to turn an ankle or tweak my knee again almost immediately. It wasn't enjoyable in any way anymore and I had to make a decision whether to carry on or to change my focus and try to develop in another area, or a different sport.

At the same time, everyone in my school was getting ready to go to university. It was the done thing: you get your GCSEs, then you get your A-levels and then you go to a university for three years. A lot of the last few months of school were dedicated to where you were going to go and what you were going to study.

My dad wasn't a huge fan of going to university for the sake of it, as you might imagine. If I had been really academic and wanted to become a doctor, that might have been different. But he and I didn't want to waste three years and get in debt, just to do a load of partying. He had no higher schooling and was a very successful businessman, so it simply didn't make sense to us. So I chose to leave education at 18 but I still wasn't sure quite what I wanted to do.

Despite my rugby career not coming to fruition, my mentality was that I was going to have a career in sport anyway and I wasn't going to let the hurdle of dodgy ankles derail my career in a physical field altogether. I had come from that background of being overweight as a young child and knew exactly how good it felt to get into better shape and I felt a connection with fitness, so I decided to become a personal trainer. Not just a regular PT. I wanted to be the biggest and best-known trainer around and then open my own gym.

Like I did when I started getting fitter, I began taking small steps to lead me to my goal. Stage one was to get the qualifications I needed, so I signed up for a one-year course at Loughborough College. I had classes twice a week and, in the meantime, I was one of the few people who got a personal training job while I was studying, starting at a Nuffield Health centre halfway through the PT course.

I fell in love with getting people fit. To look at me, you would have thought that I was a 19-year-old who had always been in good condition but on my PT advertisement I put a picture of me as a kid and a picture of me as I was at that time and it really struck a chord with people. I could empathise with clients about their journey and I got a lot of business as a result. It was hard work but the combination of my story, a laid-back attitude and the business sense that Dad had passed down to me meant that I was soon one of the busiest trainers.

I worked there for four years and became the most successful PT out of all the Nuffield Health centres in the Midlands. The managers thought I was great; I had a laugh and got on really well with everyone, but inside I wanted more. The

Start Where Others Stop mindset was now crystallising and I couldn't settle for being the best PT in that gym – I had to do something more, something bigger. I told my boss I was going to leave and start up on my own; he thought I was crazy and made the argument that I had over 40 sessions a week at the time and I wasn't going to be able to take those clients with me. But the gym was taking 50 per cent of the money I made and I knew there was much more that I could achieve, that this was just a step towards my wider goal of having my own business and a successful career in fitness.

I started a tiny personal training studio out of my parent's house. Overnight, I went from training over 40 clients a week at Nuffield to just four. But my parents had built their own business from nothing and put in some hard work at the beginning so they couldn't have been more supportive. My dad loved that I was trying to make something on my own and told me that if I needed anything, he and my mum would do their best to help.

I named it Fitness Box because the space I was running it out of was so small, then went off to the print shop and ran off hundreds and hundreds of leaflets. My mum, bless her, spent the next day driving me around while I jumped out and leafleted everywhere. We did it for a whole day, stopping at every house and block of flats in the areas around Tur Langton. I got one phone call back. We were driving around and hopping in and out of the car for eight or nine hours and I got one single call from a lady at a village church.

If it sounds to you like I'd thrown away a very secure job and set myself up for a fall, you're not the only one. All of my former colleagues at Nuffield, the manager, even some of my friends thought the same and told me I was mad, yet not a single part of me felt like it wouldn't work out. I had a goal of creating my own business in fitness and I was working towards it – whatever happened, whatever bumps or hurdles I met along the way, I would navigate them and keep moving. If you focus on the negatives, on all the little things that could go wrong, you won't get anywhere. You won't even start.

When you do hit a snag, you have to try not to be afraid to fail. It's hard, because when something doesn't work out it can feel like the end of the world, like your dream is out of reach. But it's not. Failure is nothing to be scared of, it's just a chance to learn and adapt your strategy or add in new steps towards your ultimate target. My goal then was to open my own gym and the first rung on that ladder was to reach more people. Doing one-on-one personal training was good but there was of course only one of me and I was limited by how many hours a week I could work. So I pivoted my business to concentrate on group classes instead. I changed the name to Be Fitter with the aim to start running a few group sessions to increase my profits.

BREAK DOWN FEARS

Worries, anxieties and fears are completely normal. If you have set yourself a challenging goal, addressing some or all of those anxieties may be part and parcel of the process, even of the goal itself. The simplest way to break down fears is to step back and consider what they can teach you. Why are you worried? When do the worries rise up? What do you tell yourself in those moments?

Finally, take a quick moment to appreciate your courage. Each time you consider your fears with this mindset is a step towards mastering them. Write down one of your fears in your notebook now. Say it aloud. What frightens you most about this thought? What can you do to make it seem less scary? Suddenly you'll find that you've switched to a practical way of thinking instead of being ruled by the emotional response of being scared.

My first group came from the lady at the village church, the one phone call I received after dropping off hundreds of flyers. That conversation led to a class for some of the women in the village. I ended up running that class every week for years. They loved it and so did I. Soon after, a friend and I went to a session held in the sports hall at Leicester University and it was absolutely rammed. There were 50–60 people, all paying £3.50 to be there. It seemed like a great idea, so I went around lots of different schools and leisure centres to find out how much it was to rent each space. I booked four different sports halls covering Mondays, Tuesdays, Thursdays and Saturdays every week, excited to grow my own classes as fast as possible.

I asked some loyal clients from my time at Nuffield and the few I'd picked up working for myself to come along just to bulk the numbers a bit. But it was still a *very* slow start. I remember rocking up to host a Tuesday night session where just one person came. After paying for the space, I was actually making a loss.

After a month, I was getting three people coming to the sessions. After two months, it was still only six or seven. I would drive around in my Peugeot 206 with loads of kettlebells in the boot, burning through fuel and breaking myself sometimes for a class of only a few people. Still I believed, truly believed, that new people would come to try it out if I kept plugging away. If I focused on making every session as good as it could possibly be, they would come back and they'd bring a friend or two when they did.

A few months later, I was cramming 20 people into a tiny sports hall every Tuesday night and there were always about 10 more on the waiting list. Then Thursdays got really busy too, so I started renting a bigger space to squeeze in more people and started to struggle to manage the sheer number of people in each class. Wayne – a member who absolutely loved the sessions – offered to give me a hand, so he became my first Be Fitter trainer and, with that, my business was officially larger than just me.

Then things really took off. People could pay when they turned up for classes but I was also offering memberships, so for £45 a month you could do any of the sessions you wanted. In our heyday, we got 55–60 people in a class and other PTs were always asking me how I was doing it. The real game changer was that I invented unique classes that were totally different to any that were running elsewhere, and I didn't mind telling them as I knew they probably couldn't compete.

I dreamt up this session for Saturdays called Intensity x3, a combination of spinning, kettlebells and bodyweight moves. We would mix it up a bit every week but it was brutal. We did 10 minutes of kettlebells and bodyweight and then jump on the bike for 20 minutes of sprints and steady hill climbs. Or alternated between two minutes of kettlebell swings, two minutes of burpees and two minutes of hard work on the bike. It lasted 90 minutes, so we'd end up absolutely battered by the end.

It became a massively popular class in Leicester. We had a booking system that went live at midday on a Monday and by five minutes past we were always fully booked. Other gyms started trying to copy our style of training but we'd already become known as the boys who invented these awesome classes so we were always rammed. We started doing another class on Tuesdays and that was packed out, too. Be Fitter was renowned for running the best fitness classes in the county.

It was a really satisfying period of my life. I was always pushing for more, setting goals and taking small steps to make the classes and the business as successful as possible and I wouldn't settle. If I had three packed-out halls, I wanted five. Reaching 40 members meant I wanted 50, then 60, then 100. I wanted different types of class, the best sessions and more hard-core workouts, so I researched what other people were doing and aspired to get to their standard. Then, when I believed I had, I immediately looked at someone at the next level and started doing what I could to catch up and overtake them. Be Fitter just kept growing and growing.

CHECK YOUR PROGRESS

Establishing a goal and starting to take one or two positive steps can have more of an impact than you think. If you wrote down your goal and made a note of your motivations in Chapter One, go back and look over them. How far have you come already? Even at this early stage, you might be surprised by your progress.

If your goal was to eat a healthy diet, perhaps your last supermarket shop was markedly based more around fresh fruit and vegetables. Or if you wanted to become fitter, maybe you've been out for a jog three times a week. Writing down the steps you've successfully taken is solid proof that you can achieve great things.

It was at this point that my sister became involved. I was very good at coming up with the workouts and coaching the classes and I was as fit as anything. But I was awful with all the logistics. Martine started taking care of the organisation and finances, tracking people who had paid and who owed us money. I was, from a business perspective, absolutely terrible! If somebody who had been coming to our classes for a while came up to me and told me they hadn't settled their membership yet, I would just tell them not to worry about it and that they could still jump in and train. When my sister came on board it was an immediate shift and if people didn't pay, they couldn't work out. Thanks to her, we became a really well-run business behind the scenes. We had this huge community of people who loved the classes and had all bonded over the years and we even hosted massive social events – we had 130 people turn up for one of our Christmas parties once. It was brilliant!

Alongside the classes, we started running crazy challenge days to bring people together and push the boundaries of what they thought they could achieve. The first one was called Please Call 999. It was 100 reps of nine exercises, finishing with 99 burpees. It took us about an hour to complete and afterwards everyone was buzzing with adrenaline and couldn't believe how much they'd just got done. As a result, we started doing this sort of event every three months and the members would look forward to them and train towards the different challenges. We'd finish these massive workouts then all go for food together afterwards and the feeling was infectious. They'd tell their friends about it at work or in the pub and we'd have all these new people turn up to our next sessions.

The biggest challenge we ever took on was a burpee marathon that we did for charity at Welford Road, the Leicester Tigers' stadium. We worked in teams of four and you had to do a burpee and then jump forwards, slowly racking up all the miles as we went round and round the pitch. One of you would burpee for about 200 metres while the other three walked with you and then somebody else would swap in, on and on, lap after lap. We ticked off the burpees in each segment and took it one lap at a time. Nobody looks at something like a marathon or a triathlon and thinks, 'Sure, that looks OK, I'll just do it.' You break it down into small parts that you can mentally digest or you wouldn't be able to physically handle it.

It took us 33 hours to burpee 26.2 miles. We had worked non-stop for nearly a day and a half, doing burpees in puddles under the floodlights at 3 a.m. and everyone was ruined. We raised nearly £3,000 and we were on the local news and in the papers. But more than anything, it was a huge achievement for us as the team we'd built through Be Fitter. When you've been working out constantly for over a day and you're still able to drag yourself on, hitting your burpees in the pouring rain at 5 a.m., you need that community.

It wasn't lost on me that I'd made it to the Leicester Tigers' stadium after all. Only a few years ago, I had been fully committed to the dream of going professional and playing in that stadium in front of thousands of fans every weekend. I was taking the right steps and hitting the goals I needed to in order to progress through the ranks but my injury-prone ankles and knees were something I couldn't push through. Instead, I had put in the rungs I needed to keep climbing and then taken them steadily one at a time. I had arrived at the top of the ladder all the same.

When you take your larger goal and break it into smaller steps, it means that not a single one is ever wasted. When I had to face the reality that my body could not match my drive to be a professional rugby player, all the progress I'd made up to that point set me up for success in the training industry. I had turned myself around physically, transforming myself from an overweight kid to a slightly chubby young teenager and then into somebody known by everyone as being really fit and strong who excels on the pitch. The path that I had walked meant I could genuinely connect with anyone starting out on their own fitness journey. They believed in me and my training because I had lived it. They would spend a day and a half with me doing burpees in the rain.

If you set yourself a goal and then take it one step at a time, you won't fall down. It's easy to see the setbacks you suffer along the way in a negative light and that's to be expected. If you're trying to get in shape and have been ticking off every session diligently but then miss a few because you're too busy and accidentally follow that with a big blowout at the weekend, it can feel like you weren't ever going to succeed anyway. Like giving up is the sensible option. But when you use the Start Where Others Stop mindset, each step is simply an opportunity to adapt your plan and then get back up to speed, to understand what step to take next. To figure out why you missed those gym sessions and decided to work out at a different time of day, or seeing a big weekend as giving your body a break before getting back to it with fresh motivation.

I was 22 years old and felt like I could achieve anything. Be Fitter was a massive success with a great financial model and an amazing community. It was hugely satisfying and I loved the feeling of having built it up from nothing, of starting off with a phone call from that lady at the village church.

At the same time, though, while I adored every aspect of it, the PT course and the group fitness sessions were always stepping stones. My bigger goal, the dream I had been working towards with every one of my brand-new workout classes, larger venues and crazy challenges, was to open my own gym. All I needed to do was to take it one step at a time.

SWOS PROGRAMME

In this next part of your personal Start Where Others Stop plan, we are going to work on refining your goals and establishing the micro-goals that will help you get there. When you take into account any first steps you've already taken, it's quite possible that you've exceeded your expectations by this stage. That's fine and a good sign that you need to consider your goal on a more granular level.

We're going to look at your goals under three headings. Again, fill in the exercises at the back of the book or make a few notes if you can as it will help crystallise your thoughts and give you a record to come back to when you're further along in the process.

BE PRECISE

Write down again what you want to achieve. But this time, be as detailed as you possibly can, taking in anything you have already learned from the programme and your own progress. So instead of an imprecise goal such as 'get a promotion', perhaps it might be 'become the most respected person in my company'. Note down exactly how you can measure your success and track your milestones, for example, how many clients you're going to bring in before the year end.

BE CHALLENGED

Push yourself a bit outside of your comfort zone. This is the perfect time to evaluate the goals you've set yourself. If your goal is challenging, you are going to be more motivated and excited about making it happen and your end target should be ambitious but attainable, if you take the right steps. Too general and it will be harder to stay the course. Simply saying you're going to get better at running isn't enough but set your sights on a good time for a ten-kilometre run though and you're in the perfect zone.

BE CLEAR

Complexity is the enemy of daily improvement, so break your larger goal into chunks. If you want to work towards a healthier weight, let's say you set yourself the target of burning off two kilograms by the end of the month. Then split that down into smaller segments. In this example it would be four weeks, so you could set yourself the mini-goal of exercising five times per week. Then break it down into days: what can you do on a daily basis to contribute to your weekly and monthly goals? Getting to bed early so you can go for a run first thing, perhaps. Or maybe eating a healthy breakfast so you are less likely to snack mid-morning.

Break down your end goal into mini- and micro-goals and keep those notes to hand, either on your phone or on a piece of paper where you can see them. Having those shorter-term and mid-term items to tick off will keep you moving on an upward curve without having to worry about the high-level ambition. That will take care of itself.

CHAPTER THREE

PURSUE YOUR PASSION

If you've ever had to do something fairly difficult that did not interest you on any level, you will know how much of a slog it is to get it done. The whole thing drags from the very start and each step towards completion is increasingly hard to take, which only stretches out the process even further. It's a grind.

'Grinding' has become a popular term recently and when it's used to mean giving your best at work every day, or resolutely chipping away at a DIY project around the house, then embracing the grind can be a positive thing. However, if it's used to describe the drag of pursuing something that you are not excited about, then it is a dangerous misconception that can see you listlessly plugging away for the sake of it. If you can align your goals with your interests, you won't have to grind half as much and, when you do, you will have more than enough internal motivation to power through and pick up the pace again.

We opened the doors to Be Fitter Gym in 2014. That day was a huge milestone for me and something that I'd been driving towards with everything I had since I started my PT course after leaving school. In all those classes, from one person turning up, to packing out massive sports halls with 60 members all paying us a monthly fee, the goal was always to have our own space and to make it a success. I understood how to build something up from nothing and had total faith in my ability to achieve through the power of my mindset and my wholesale motivation to make things happen.

It had not been a straightforward process at all, especially as we had some issues with the council about changing the use of the space we had chosen and even parking regulations. We were back and forth with them for a whole year before opening, but we kept on pushing and it was all very exciting. There was a team of four of us who owned that gym – me, my sister Martine, Wayne (who had come on board running the classes in the sports halls) and a guy called Matt. Matt was another person who had been a regular at our classes and wanted to invest and become a part of the journey.

The first year was a lot of fun. We were pumped about it all and especially excited to be branching out and trying to cater to lots of different types of training to maximise our membership. We had loads of people join from our Be Fitter gang and saw an influx of people joining because we were a new gym. We had a big studio for the fitness classes, as they had done so well for us, and we wanted to protect the sense of community we'd worked so hard to foster, but we also had free weights and resistance machines to attract some general bodybuilding types, or people who just wanted somewhere to exercise a bit. My dream was to make that site a success and then open another one, and another. I wanted Be Fitter to become a chain of gyms, all packed to the rafters with happy members.

But after only three years, we had to close and shut the doors for good. Things didn't turn out like I planned and, no matter how hard I worked or how many new ideas I tried, I simply couldn't make it profitable. It was the first major setback I'd ever experienced. It was the first time that I had poured my heart and soul into something and found out that it wasn't enough.

I learned a crucially valuable lesson, though: if you want to reach your goal, you have to make sure it is something you are truly passionate about. I can guarantee you there will still be plenty of periods of grind along the way but it does make each stage of the journey infinitely more enjoyable. If you're doing or working towards something you care about then you can endure that grind with a smile on your face and each barrier becomes a chance to jump even higher, rather than somewhere to stumble, fall and give up. Having the drive to match your dream can work and it had worked for me up until this point. But aligning your dream with your desires is the keystone.

All you need to do is find your passion. And if one comes

along when you're least expecting it, grab hold and run with it. The three years of hard work that ended when we locked the doors of Be Fitter Gym for the last time were not wasted because I had found my passion. I had found CrossFit.

FIND YOUR WHY

Why do you want to achieve your goal? It is valid to simply want to be a better version of yourself in some way and all personal development is positive. But if you can align your goal with something you feel genuine passion and excitement for, you will be far more motivated to make it happen.

Go back to the breakdown of mini- and micro-goals you established in the last chapter and be honest with yourself. If the daily, weekly and even monthly items are not as engaging as they should be, it is a sign that your goal may need tweaking.

In 2013, when we had just started going back and forth with the council trying to open the gym, my dad showed me a video from the recent CrossFit Games. This is the culmination of the competitive season, with an elite group of men, women and teams vying for the title of 'Fittest on Earth', representing the top 0.001 per cent, who are often referred to as 'the tip of the spear'. To make it to the Games even once marks you out as a supreme athlete with a huge range of capacities and skills.

I didn't know any of that at the time, though I will always remember that video. It was of an event called 'The Pool', which featured swimming and bar muscle-ups, where you have to propel your body up to and over a pull-up bar. There was a shot of the three top athletes, Ricgh Froning Jr, Jason Khalipa and Matt Chan, lining up before they walked out for the event. They looked absolutely jacked. When they all dived into the pool then started jumping out and busting out muscle-ups, I was instantly hooked. I had no idea what they were doing or why they were doing it. But I knew I wanted to do it too.

I went online, found a CrossFit gym in Northampton, called them up and went along the next day. For most of 2013, while I was waiting to open Be Fitter Gym, I was driving 45–50 minutes twice a week, having an hour one-on-one session with one of the coaches there called Greg, then trekking home again. It was taking me three hours just for a workout but I was enjoying learning all the techniques and skills involved in the sport. I wanted to get into competing almost immediately and they were really helpful with signing me up for local events. After only two months of CrossFit training, I entered my first competition, Battle for the Midlands.

I stayed at my sister's flat the night before, as she lived in

Northampton at the time. I was so nervous that I couldn't sleep and I didn't want to eat anything for breakfast in the morning. When I registered and walked into the athletes' warm-up area, I felt like the newbie that I truly was, so I just sat quietly in one corner. All of the more experienced athletes were sharing barbells while warming up and taking it in turns on the pieces of gymnastic equipment but I couldn't do many of the technical gymnastic movements and I didn't want to show myself up in front of everyone, so I just sat waiting until a barbell was free and then used it quickly in case anyone thought I was hogging it.

Looking back, I just wanted someone to talk to me and say, 'Yeah, this one is going to be all right, isn't it?' Now that I'm an experienced, elite athlete, if I see somebody looking nervous before an event, I always go up and talk to them, make sure they're all right and ask them how they feel about the next workout. Though at least I was there with a friend of mine, Josh, who was also competing for the first time. We were mates but obviously we wanted to beat each other and that probably made us go even harder than we would have done otherwise.

I was doing quite well and was in the main heat with the other top-ranked athletes. The next event was a 'chipper' – a workout with a huge number of repetitions that you have to 'chip' away at. There were sets of 40, 30, 20 and 10 toes-to-ring – which means hanging by your hands from a pair of Olympic rings then using your abs to bring your feet up to touch the rings. I had no idea how to do them but I saw other people practising before the beginning of the workout and reckoned I'd be all right. I watched as everyone in the heats before me did each set of toes-to-ring without taking a break. So, obviously, I tried to do mine unbroken, too.

On that very first movement, I totally redlined, which is when your muscles are so fatigued that you are practically incapable of continuing. I did 30 reps keeping up with everyone else but then had to do the last 10 one-by-one, dropping down from the rings each time. And this was the *start* of the workout. It only went downhill from there. My family were in the crowd right next to me and were screaming at me that I just needed to jump back up to the rings and keep going but I physically couldn't and could only shake my head at them, saying 'I can't! My abs are cramping up!' By the end of the competition, I had torn most of the skin on my hands and I ended up finishing twenty-first overall.

I had felt good on the basic fitness work, like the burpees and rowing, and, although my barbell lifting was terrible, I was big and strong enough to manhandle the weights. But the technical gymnastics and the lifting technique were far beyond me then. I remember so many people saying 'Oh, you're a big lad, aren't you?' and I don't think they expected me to go far in the sport just because the top athletes in the sport tend to be a good bit shorter and much lighter than I am. I'm certainly not a typical CrossFit shape.

It's cool to think back to that first competition and how

everything felt, the sense of the unknown and a stomach full of nerves; having no idea how to pace or attack a workout and not even being able to do every movement. Despite all of that, I already knew that this was the sport for me. I looked at the winner that weekend, a guy called Mitch Adams, and I wanted to get to that level. I wanted to be better than that. When I got home, I wrote 'make the CrossFit Games' on a piece of paper and stuck it to a board hanging on my bed-room wall. I've still got that same goals board today.

When we finally opened Be Fitter Gym in 2014, I no longer had time to make the trip up to Northampton to train twice a week. Instead, I installed a little CrossFit rig with everything I needed to train in the corner of the gym. We used to open at 6 a.m. and close at 10 p.m. and I'd be there all day. It was fun but a lot of extremely hard work and I was doing seven or eight hours of one-on-one personal training a day to try and bring in as much money as possible, while also trying to work out myself as much as I could every single day. I would do four PT sessions in the morning, squeeze in my CrossFit for an hour at 1 p.m., take another three or four clients in the afternoon, do a second CrossFit workout and then teach the late class in the evening. That was how every day went, Monday to Friday. At the weekend we weren't open quite as much, so I'd just train more and really punish myself with longer, gruelling sessions.

Obviously, with such a brutal daily schedule, I wasn't

getting much better and I certainly was not improving at the rate I had imagined I would. But back then, I thought the solution was simply to go harder, practise as much as possible and train with more intensity. I was poring over every CrossFit-related video on YouTube and trying to match my level of training to the elite athletes in all the documentaries. My theory then was that if Rich Froning Jr worked out three times a day for hours at a time, then I should too if I wanted to get to the top of the sport. I was qualifying for some fairly large UK events and travelling around the country to compete. At the time, I was just chuffed to be there, although my ability as an athlete wasn't improving fast enough, regardless of how hard I pushed myself.

Every week and month that went by while we were grafting away to try to make Be Fitter Gym a success, I was becoming progressively more obsessed with CrossFit. In an effort to diversify, we'd lost the community vibe we had when we were doing the classes and were trying to attract your everyday gym goer, even though we weren't a gym specifically tailored to that sort of person. Meanwhile, I was spending more and more time crushing myself on the little rig in my corner.

That's when I met Harmeet Singh. He came into the gym just to train in 2015, when we'd been open for a year and a half or so. Harmeet walking into Be Fitter was a big turning point for me. He was a certified CrossFit coach who had just moved over from Dubai and he spotted me training in the corner and could tell straight away from the clothes and shoes I was wearing that I was into CrossFit. Harmeet saw me strict shoulder pressing a 100kg barbell, walked over and said, 'You're strong, dude!'

We started chatting and I told him that my goal was to compete at the CrossFit Games. He could see I had out-and-out strength but asked me to show him some gymnastics. I could just about do butterfly pull-ups – a method of doing pull-ups that uses the power of your hips and lower body to help you speed through reps when you're trying to go as fast as possible in a workout. That was the most technical thing I could manage. Harmeet said he would coach me: we'd get to the CrossFit Games and that we'd get there together. And that was it.

TELL SOMEONE ABOUT IT

Once you have successfully set your objectives, sharing them with a person you trust will enhance your progress. A study conducted at Dominican University, Illinois recruited 267 business people and divided them into five groups. The first set no goals and had no concrete plans. The second group set goals but did not prepare a plan. The third group prepared well-defined goals and plans of action. The fourth had detailed goals and plans, then sent them to a friend. The fifth group prepared their goals and plans, then sent them to a friend, as well as checking in with them to provide weekly progress reports.

The final group achieved notably more progress than all of the other groups, which proves the efficacy of writing down your goals while also planning the smaller wins that will get you there. Telling somebody about your plan and how you're progressing will let you use the psychological tools of commitment and accountability to significantly boost your motivation. Who can you tell today about your goal?

We trained together pretty much every day. Harmeet taught me all my initial gymnastic movements; we worked on my mobility and drilled the big Olympic lifts, which are the snatch and the clean and jerk. In the snatch, you pull the bar from the ground and catch it overhead with straight arms with one movement, so it's very technical. On the clean and jerk you receive the bar across the front of your shoulders first, then 'jerk' it over your head, which means you can generally go a bit heavier. Harmeet was very inspirational; I looked up to him for all the movements he could do. Now we laugh about some of the workouts we did back then, but at the time we thought were absolute ninjas! The first time I did 30 muscle-ups it took me 29 minutes to finish all the reps. Now my record is two minutes!

Even though I was a long, long way from being good enough to qualify for the CrossFit Games, training with Harmeet was making a big difference to my overall ability.

More importantly, my focus had started to shift and I increasingly felt like I wanted to dedicate more time to being an athlete, rather than being caught up in the daily grind of trying to make the business work. I just wasn't passionate about it anymore.

CHANGE FOR THE BETTER

If your goals are long term, they will change in some way in the process of working towards them. That change is good, it is a natural result of developing and refining your ability to set clear goals and take the correct steps to achieving them. It is only to be expected that, sometimes, your experience shows you that your original goal wasn't quite right.

Read through your original goals you wrote down at the very start of this book and take a minute to think about how you could adapt that ambition based on the knowledge you've gained so far. It could be that you've found a new goal that has absorbed all your attention. Perhaps you just need to alter the timeframe you imagined for yourself. Embrace the change and move forwards.

Be Fitter Gym was a goal that I had worked towards for

so long and it had been such a slog even to get to a point of opening the doors. But you have to be totally committed to cover your overheads and make as much money as you can when you own a gym. You have to deal with members cancelling and not telling you, or direct debits bouncing. You'd think that if we had 700 members all paying a membership, we would have been rolling in cash. But the gym itself just swallowed most of it up. The rent, business rates, utilities and even upkeep of the equipment left the four us taking home only about £1,000 each a month. It was unsustainable but we had all given everything we had, pushing through those endless weeks of 12 to 14-hour days, so we had been ignoring the warning signs.

After three years of operation, the number of members simply wasn't getting to the level we needed it to be in order to make any sort of profit with four people in a business and those overheads were killing us. Around this time, my sister wanted to start a family. When Martine became pregnant, the direction of her life obviously changed. She had been fully focused on making the gym as good as it could be but when she realised she was having a kid, she needed to do something else and make some proper money. She wanted to give her child the best possible life. Meanwhile, it was understandably becoming a real issue for Wayne and Matt that, despite all our work, we still weren't making any money.

The direction of my life was changing, too. I wanted to be a full-time CrossFit athlete and commit myself entirely to my goal of getting to the Games and that just wasn't going to happen with the insane amount of hours it took to run a business that was struggling to stay afloat.

For the last half a year or so, it was obvious the business wasn't going the right way but I still thought I might be able to turn it round, or if we changed a few things it could work. We knew deep down, however, that we would probably have to close and we talked endlessly about the right time to tell the members and how much notice to give people, while I carried on wracking my brains for a new marketing idea or a new class that would pull in extra members. Looking back on it now, we were just putting off the inevitable.

In the end, we came to a decision when one day I woke up and said to myself, 'I'm going to shut it.' I told my sister and we stuck a sign on the door saying, 'Sorry. We're closed' and that was that. After all the build-up and strategising, we just stuck a sign on the door with some sticky tape.

It was the first time I had set myself a goal, achieved that goal but then things had not gone to plan and I found it a very hard pill to swallow. It felt like the worst thing that could ever happen to me. After locking the doors for the last time, I sat in my car and cried down the phone to my dad. Having been in business his whole life, Dad had been up and down four or five times and nearly gone bankrupt, even. If you talk to any successful business person, they will probably have the same sort of stories. I felt like I had failed massively but he reminded me that everything hadn't always gone smoothly for him, either. He gave me the pep talk I needed that night. He said, 'Zack, you haven't failed and nobody in business is a success first time. You've got to use this as a chance to work out what direction you want to go in next, that's all. This can be a positive opportunity if you want it to be.' He was brilliant.

Dad knew I was really into CrossFit and I already thought that I wanted to open a CrossFit gym. Not with the goal of making it extremely successful and starting my own chain this time – instead I wanted to get back to the community we had when we did the classes. I wanted a smaller gym where I didn't have to worry about all the overheads as much and I could reignite that family feel that we used to have before opening Be Fitter, when loads of us were doing burpees in the rain in the middle of the night.

More than that, though, I wanted to become the best athlete I could possibly be. So I wanted to be around people who wanted to do CrossFit and be in an environment every day that would maximise my potential, to see if I could make a career for myself as an athlete.

After I explained this to my dad, he just said, 'All right. We'll do it then.' He said that even if I felt like I'd failed, I had learned a lot and I had changed in those three years and now, aged 26, my career was just taking a different path. He told me that I hadn't failed at all; I just needed to adjust slightly and then crack on.

He was right, of course. He was bang on, as mums and

dads normally are. You have to adjust your goals if your situation changes. My goal had always been to have a successful career in the fitness industry, it's just that the passion I had for competing, my ambition to make it to the CrossFit Games had altered my direction of travel.

Dad told me that as soon as we'd finished on the phone, I should book a two-week holiday, so I could relax and chill out about everything. He said he would give me some money so that I wouldn't have to worry and could just de-stress as much as possible, and that we would devise a plan for a CrossFit gym when I got back.

It was the best advice I could have been given at the time. So many other people would have said that it was hard luck about the 'whole gym thing' and would have told me to get a normal job, but my dad's attitude, the way he'd brought us up, was exactly what I needed. It was the mental boost I required, to make me see that pursuing my passion was not just the right thing to do, it was the *only* thing I should do. That there was no doubting that at all.

I went to Crete for two weeks and sat on the beach and by the pool. It was the space I craved from the madness that was the final throes of Be Fitter but my mind was already busy thinking about the new gym. In the course of that fortnight, I pretty much worked out every single aspect of how it would come together, what equipment we'd need, what the timetable would be, the names of all the classes, the initial start-up costs, the monthly overheads and the membership fees. I had

90 per cent of it designed before even getting on the plane home.

As soon as I got back, I called Harmeet and asked him if he wanted to open the gym with me. I planned to ask Dad for a loan, so I said I would fund everything to start with and then we'd go 50–50, but I told him that, at some point when the time was right, he would have to handle all the coaching so I could become a full-time athlete. Harmeet said, 'Great! Let's do it!'

Those first few weeks after my holiday was the first time I had really stopped and evaluated what was going on, actually sat down and thought, really thought, about what I was excited by and why. The previous three years had been such an endless grind but I wouldn't change it for the world. It added another crucial aspect to my mental strength and I learned that overcoming a hurdle sometimes means taking a slightly different route. If you then go in a direction in which you feel fully invested, you're headed the right way.

Even though I wanted to dedicate myself to my training, I still needed the gym to work financially. Some of my friends thought I was crazy for opening another gym right around the corner from the one I'd just closed but I'd learned so much from the last three years. It wasn't that Be Fitter wasn't busy or popular – we were one of the busiest independent gyms in Leicester and we won best newcomer at the National Fitness Awards in 2016 – I just had my calculations wrong.

The premises I was interested in was much cheaper in

terms of rent and had better business rates, so instead of having to aim for 800 members, we now only needed 150 to make decent money. It would have been easy, perhaps even more sensible, to have given up on the fitness industry at this point and settled into an office job, but I would not have been passionate about it in the slightest. It would have sucked the life out of me.

I consider myself incredibly fortunate to have the support of such amazing parents. For them to not only have my back but at the same time bring me up to work hard, to set goals and make my own way, is something I'm thankful for every day. Now I also knew that it doesn't matter if you fail so long as you learn. Dad would have openly told me I was completely stupid if I'd opened up a new gym and made exactly the same mistakes as I did the first time around. Instead, he saw that I had adapted and, crucially, that I was passionate, borderline obsessive, in fact, about my new path.

So, he fronted me the money to cover all the start-up costs and, within two months of the first gym closing, we opened CrossFit BFG. It was only about a one-minute walk from the old location, so we walked over all the kit we needed. Loads of our original members came to help and 12 of us picked up the rig we'd had in the corner and carried it down the road to the new place. It's still there today.

I was a stone's throw away from a business that I had been forced to shut down and it had only been a few weeks since I got back from being on the beach but it felt like a million miles away from that first gym. It felt like a place where I could develop into the person I now knew I wanted to become: a professional CrossFit athlete who would compete at the CrossFit Games. It felt like home and we're still here. Two years later, I had paid Dad back in full.

The CrossFit Open is an annual online competition that is the first stage of qualification for the CrossFit Games. Anyone in the world can register to compete across five workouts, with one announced per week for five weeks. The details of each workout are kept secret until the Friday and then you get until the Monday to register your best score. You have your attempt judged and verified by a coach with an official qualification from CrossFit or, failing that, you can film yourself completing the workouts and send the videos in. At the top level of the sport, athletes must both have their workouts judged and submit films for further scrutiny by CrossFit HQ. One second or a single rep can make a vital difference to your total score.

The first year I entered the Open was 2016, when I was still working every hour I could to try to keep our first gym afloat. I didn't complete all five workouts as I couldn't do all the movements but I finished three out of the five and it gave me a clear idea of where I needed to improve.

The following year, in 2017, I finished every Open workout. After the five weeks, I was 970th in the world, out of over 20,000 male athletes who registered. I was happy to have completed all the work but it was only a few months before we had to shut Be Fitter and I was getting absolutely battered with work stuff left, right and centre. Mentally, I was distracted by the fact that the business was doing really badly and I was just trying to do too much and juggle too many balls. We all know that, whether you're trying to excel on the sports field, at home or in the office, if you're stressed or you feel mentally unbalanced, it's going to seriously hinder your performance.

Harmeet and I had been hard at work, concentrating on my gymnastics, weightlifting and pretty much anything technical so both my strength and now my fitness were now good. But it wasn't until we opened CrossFit BFG that we started to tap into my real potential. When we first started, we split the coaching, so even though I was doing much less than I was at the Be Fitter Gym, I was still not able to devote as much of myself as an athlete as I wanted to.

By the time we'd been up and running a year or so, we had got the situation sorted. Harmeet was covering a lot of the classes and, a while later, a member, Josh Burniston, qualified as a coach and joined the team full time. Josh had never tried CrossFit before he became a member and I found out not long ago that he was very near to quitting after a couple of weeks because he couldn't get the hang of the technique for butterfly pull-ups. Two years later, he's our main coach and he absolutely loves it.

BEING SELFISH IS OK

Committing yourself to any form of individual goal can sometimes feel like a selfish pursuit. After all, you are setting yourself a target and working out what you need to do in order to hit your smaller goals along your way, so it is inherently about you. But you can take steps to limit any guilt by reflecting on how your personal betterment can have a positive effect on other people.

Research published in the journal *Annual Review of Psychology* states that receiving support of some sort actually improves relationships, brings you closer to those helping you and fosters commitment, trust and even intimacy.

Speak to three people close to you, whether that's your partner, your friends, your family or even your colleagues, and ask them how they feel about your commitment to your goal. Ask them what they have noted so far and how they imagine you achieving your dream would impact them. Odds are that you will find out how focusing on yourself more imparts wider benefits on the people around you. Happiness breeds happiness. Don't lose sight of that.

We didn't have to worry about advertising to bring in new people because we had developed a very good, stable membership base. I remember feeling like the business was taking care of itself, we had amazing coaches and a fantastic community. Now was the time for me to focus fully on getting to the Games. I called Harmeet one night to tell him that I thought it was the right moment for me to take a step back and he couldn't have been more supportive. He and Josh took care of everything from that point and I dedicated myself to training.

In the year before the 2018 CrossFit Open I all but stopped working, only covering the odd class here or there, probably less than 15 per cent of how much I was coaching in 2017. I had been doing the sport for that little bit longer now and was becoming exponentially more efficient with my movements as a result. With Josh and Harmeet covering the day-to-day running of the gym, though, the real benefit was how much I was able to concentrate on my recovery. Instead of teaching the 6.15 a.m. class three times a week and getting six hours of sleep, I was now logging nine hours a night. You can't under-estimate how much difference getting the adequate amount of sleep makes, as an athlete, or as a person simply trying to feel healthier, more energetic and on top of things.

So I was recovering from workouts much more quickly as a result. I could come in mid-morning, focus properly on stretching and mobility and then hit my training session, then go home to have some food and maybe sleep a bit, or just chill out. I would head back to the gym for my second session later in the afternoon before going back home again to eat dinner, relax and go to bed. I was, at last, living my life as a professional athlete.

Sticking that sign up on Be Fitter Gym that said we were closing down had felt like the door had slammed shut on my ambitions. But the more I was drawn to the little rig in the corner and the competitive drive that was accelerating with each local event or CrossFit Open workout had been early signs of the thirst I had already developed for the sport. It was unquenchable.

Making it to the CrossFit Games had been on that board on my bedroom wall for over four years by this point and even though I realised it was a massive goal, I could see that there was a clear process and path of development. Most importantly, the passion I had to get there was without question. I thought about it every single day, picturing jogging out into packed arenas alongside the most elite athletes in the world, about becoming a part of the top 0.001 per cent and reaching the tip of the spear.

To achieve my dream, to tick off that goal that had started when I watched that video of the CrossFit Games in 2013, I had to finish in the top 20 in the Central European area in order to qualify for Regionals. That was the next step. I just needed to reach for it.

YOUR SWOS PROGRAMME

Now that you are well underway with your goal setting, the last task in the first section of your programme is to evaluate your progress and ensure your goal is aligned with something you are truly passionate about.

Let's say you want to reach a particular level in your company, or to bring in a certain amount of money a year. You could dedicate yourself to knuckling down and grafting away to reach that status or earn that salary. But unless there is a deeper reason for the hard work, you will get burned out. We are all much more motivated by what we feel, so achievements are infinitely more attainable if it is something that feels important to us.

For this last stage of the first part of the Start Where Others Stop journey, you're going to draw a line down a piece of paper to make two columns. In one, write 'How will I feel when I achieve my goal?' and in the other, write 'How will I feel if I don't achieve my goal?' Alternatively, head to page 232 where there's a table ready for you to fill in.

Start making notes in each column, focusing always on how you will feel.

HOW WILL I FEEL WHEN I ACHIEVE MY GOAL?

If you answer with positive and excited feelings then it is a sign you are passionate about your direction. If you know that you would be happier in another career, say, or feel real contentment moving your family into a new home, then you will find it easier to switch lanes professionally or save in the long-term to buy a new house.

HOW WILL I FEEL IF I DON'T ACHIEVE MY GOAL?

If you answer that you will be upset, disappointed and unhappy, those are also signs that you're passionate about your goal. If you tend towards phrases like 'I wouldn't be too bothered' or 'I would get over it', there is likely a disconnection between your feelings and your ambitions. If so, you are free to adapt your goal or to choose one that you are more passionate about. This is something to strongly consider.

If your goal is one that you need to achieve, irrespective of being entirely excited about it – a work project for example – then you need to find ways to make that process more enjoyable. Maybe there are valuable things you can learn from the experience that will give it more meaning, or you can find ways to make each step of the process more engaging.

PART II

OVERCOME CHALLENGES

CHAPTER FOUR

COMMIT TO THE MOMENT

It comes off like a wellness cliché to 'be present' but you don't have to sit in silence with your legs crossed. My mindfulness is training in the gym and competing is my meditation. When you're in the middle of a workout and pushing yourself to be your best, all you are thinking about is the next rep – listening to every muscle in your body and sensing whether you need to take a quick break, feeling your heart beat and consciously breathing rhythmically to keep yourself calm. You are aware of the other people in the gym, or on the competition floor next to you but, at that moment, your world is that workout.

Win or lose, there is always something worth celebrating. If you have had real success, like a promotion or landing a new client, then that is obviously hugely satisfying, but if things didn't quite happen the way you thought, you can still seek the positives and look forward to improving next time. Whatever happens, spending too long looking backwards or gazing forwards means you can easily miss the joy of the here and now.

It was a lesson I learned in 2018, the first year I felt like I was developing into a half-decent athlete. I was starting to get a grasp of how to programme my own workouts, building an understanding of what I needed to focus on and I felt physically and mentally like I was ready to take the next step by qualifying for Regionals.

At the time, CrossFit had divided the world into nine separate regions. If you finished in the top 20 in your individual area, you went through to a live three-day competition with the 40 best athletes in your part of the world. Only the top five at the end of the weekend would receive an invite to the CrossFit Games, which were held each summer in Madison, Wisconsin, USA. My ultimate goal was to get to the Games but the first stage of that plan was to be good enough to qualify for the European Regional. It is a genuine honour to be able to call yourself a 'regional athlete' and it marks you out as a serious competitor.

Everyone knew my goal was to get to the CrossFit Games as it was a dream that I was not at all shy about sharing with people. After all, I told Harmeet within minutes of meeting him in the corner of the old gym! Although the goal was a massive one, I had established a clear way to make progress step by step. First I had to improve my performance in the Open in order to make it through to Regionals. After that I had to move up the Regionals leader board in subsequent years until I finished fifth or better. Then, with all that done, I would be on the plane to Madison.

In between those clear milestones were countless markers to pass in the gym: refining my skills, building on my strengths and working on my weaknesses, for hours every day, six days a week, month after month. I had to find ways to recover more effectively and perform at my best on a daily basis. I would have to make sure my environment, my routine and even the people around me were all conducive to my success.

If that sounds like hard work, it was and it still is. It's work I do with genuine happiness, though, because I relish and celebrate each milestone I reach along the way, big and small – the major competitions, obviously, but also the little wins of a really good day of training too.

If you don't let yourself take real satisfaction in your progress, if you fail to look around and see how far you've come, the rest of the road will seem to stretch far out to the horizon and beyond. You'll lose sight of why you started out on your journey and where you were aiming to get to. Your speed will slow and you'll wish you had realised there were so many places you could have stopped, taken a deep breath and really savoured the trip.

I was about to reach my first major waypoint in my new career as a CrossFit athlete: the European Regional. It was a massive milestone on my path to the CrossFit Games and one that I could have quite easily tried to speed past in an attempt to get to my destination as fast as possible. Instead,

I stopped for that moment. I took a breath, enjoyed myself and squeezed every single drop of positive energy from the experience. And I did a lot of dancing.

On my previous attempts at the Open, we were still at the commercial gym, which wasn't geared up for CrossFit at all. My little rig in the corner was just about good enough for training but couldn't handle competing in a worldwide online qualifier. I would travel around to other CrossFit boxes to do the various Open workouts and the year before I had done all five events with my mate Craig Richey at CrossFit Faber near Coventry, almost a two-hour drive away.

By the time that 2018 Open came around, we had been in CrossFit BFG for almost a year and all the good training sessions, better recovery and a lot more sleep had made a huge difference. I was logging nine hours of sleep every night, more rest between my two workouts and only doing about two hours of teaching, rather than the eight to ten I was coaching at the first gym. So everything was infinitely more conducive to performing to my full potential.

Most people underestimate how much of an advantage it is being in your usual environment and being able to keep to your normal routines when you want to be at your best. For me that year, that meant being able to sleep in my own bed and wake up in my own home on a Friday morning. My girlfriend, Sam, and I would have our normal breakfast and she would make sure I had the snacks and the food I needed before we left for the gym to attempt that week's Open workout. When we got there, I could set things up exactly how I needed it, so I wasn't wasting precious time racing around from one piece of kit to another.

I also had Ben Bodycombe, who had quickly become my 'stats' guy and his help was crucial to all the Open workouts we did that year. Ben would work out all the reps or splits I'd need to hit to get a certain score or time and then have it ready on a whiteboard so that I could keep an eye on it during the workout. I even had two people filming me to make sure we had the video in case CrossFit HQ requested the evidence. All the logistics were covered and I could just concentrate on smashing each workout as hard and fast as I could.

COVER ALL YOUR BASES

Whether in the process of working towards a goal, or simply in life in general, there will always be big days that you need to build up to. Most people would be happy simply practising a big speech or ticking off the training sessions before a half marathon. But going into more detail with your preparation will set you up for real success on the day.

We all have a tendency to imagine the best-case scenario and it's human nature to picture everything going perfectly. We do not spend enough energy figuring out what could go wrong. That is not a negative outlook, rather it allows you to plan for any eventuality and react positively in the moment. It is the true definition of preparation.

I'm going to use that half marathon as an example but the same process can be applied to any event, be that interviewing for a new role, hosting a big birthday for a loved one or taking your family away for the weekend. Simply plan as far in advance as is appropriate and consider all the possible angles.

ONE MONTH BEFORE

Get to grips with the course and, if you can, plan training runs to cover parts of it in order to dispel any confusion or distraction on the day of the race. Check previous reviews of the race online, if they are available, to get a feel for the general set up.

TWO WEEKS BEFORE

Take all your kit for a trial run. Wear the exact shoes, socks, shorts or leggings, top and any other accessories you intend to wear on the day if the weather is good. Then add or swap in any items necessary should conditions be bad. Mile six is not the time to realise that your T-shirt is chafing . . .

ONE WEEK BEFORE

Plan how you're going to get to the start line on the day. If you're going by car, work out where to park and how long it will take you to drive there, adding plenty of extra time for traffic. If you're going by public transport, check the race website for suggested routes then cross-reference those with local transport. Buy any tickets in advance if possible to save time on the day.

TWO DAYS BEFORE

If anyone is coming to cheer you on, establish a mile marker and on which side of the road they are going to be so you can spot them mid-race. Give them your bib number if you have it. Ask them to bring any extra drinks or snacks in case you can't get any at the aid stations for some reason. Or if you just need a pick me up!

The Open events are always horribly painful. It doesn't matter how strong or fit you are, they all hurt just the same. If you're a beginner in the sport, they punish you and you struggle to see how you will ever get to the end. If you're an elite athlete, they hit you in the exact same way, you just get to the end a little bit quicker.

What I hadn't realised going into that season was the impact of having my friends, family and the CrossFit BFG community there to support me and cheer me on. When you feel like you're dying halfway through a workout, support like that directly improves your performance. The fifth and last workout that year tasked you with performing as many bar-bell thrusters – going down into a full squat with the bar and then standing up and punching it straight up overhead – and chest-to-bar pull-ups as you could in seven minutes. It doesn't sound long but you're moving so fast that after two minutes your legs are like lead from the thrusters, your forearms are burning from all the pull-ups and your lungs feel like they are on fire.

Your nearest and dearest, your whole team, screaming you on when you want to stop for ten seconds to catch your breath or spend too long shaking out your arms before each set of pull-ups is incredibly motivating. The energy it gives you is impossible to replicate when you're working out on your own – nothing matches that feeling.

That last workout was my best effort that year – I came fifth in the Europe Central region. But with two scores in the mid-twenties and the other two placing me 113th and 162nd, it was going to be touch and go whether I'd made it into the top 20. I didn't care where I came so long as I had qual-ified. When everyone's scores were in, I was in nineteenth position. I had only just squeaked in. But I had made it.

It was such a massive achievement for me. It was my first, honest realisation that I could hang out with the big boys of the sport and the mental boost that reaching such a major milestone on my way to making it to the CrossFit Games was *huge*. There is no other word for that feeling. It enhanced my approach to everything, my training, my nutrition, my recovery, even how I carried myself as I walked around. I was Zack George – a CrossFit Regional athlete.

At least, I really hoped I was. Although the online leader board says you've qualified, you still have to wait for a month or so while CrossFit HQ checks and verifies all the videos to make sure you haven't missed any reps or failed to execute the movements to the required standards. If they judge that you didn't lock out your knees at the top of a few of the deadlifts, for example, or didn't get your chin above the bar on all of those pull-ups, they will adjust your results. If it's a race against the clock, they will add extra time; if it's a workout where you have to get as many reps as possible, they will deduct the reps they deem to be in breach of the regulations.

It was a stressful month waiting for the official results to come back. I was training with my friends John Chapman and Leon Bustin, at their local gym in Norwich, CrossFit Spitfire, when I finally got the email through to say that I'd qualified. One of the athletes who finished ahead of me opted to compete on a team rather than as an individual, so I was eighteenth in the end. We had a little celebration and I was over the moon. I knew, as soon as I was officially going to the European Regional, that I wanted to enjoy the experience as much as possible, to soak in every second and every moment of what it felt like to compete on that next level.

CELEBRATE TOGETHER

It's important that you feel the personal satisfaction of reaching a milestone on your journey towards your grander ambition and that is a deeply motivating force for future success. Yet to only celebrate internally is to rob yourself of the benefits of enjoying those moments with other people who understand your goal.

There is science behind this. Researchers at Brigham Young University found that sharing positive moments with others markedly increased the levels of enjoyment for all parties. In their study, positive emotions such as happiness peaked when sharing experiences and the listener gives a constructive response.

Go back to chapter three and remind yourself who you spoke to about your goal and how it made them feel. If any of those people struck you as being totally on board with your plan, then they are the sort of person you want to celebrate a big win with. It doesn't mean

> they have to be there when you reach your milestone, of course. Instead, you could go out for dinner to celebrate or even just schedule a Zoom call to chat. The important thing is to book in that time to savour the feeling with somebody else. A problem shared is a problem halved. But a victory shared is doubled.

The 2018 European Regional was held in Berlin and I flew out with John and Leon. Sam couldn't make it for the whole competition but she came for the end and about 20 people from the gym made the trip to support me too. There was a real squad of us there and it was such a brilliant atmosphere.

The Regionals are the only stage of the process at which CrossFit releases the details of some of the workouts in advance, so you can practise them ahead of the live competition. Most athletes constantly try out parts of the event so they can pick the best strategy and know when it makes sense for them to push and when they need to dial things back in order not to redline.

You'd think I would have seized this information and used it to make sure I was well rehearsed ahead of the event. However, for some reason that still confuses me today, I didn't practise *any* of the workouts. It wasn't exactly sensible, and I work tirelessly on my tactics now, but I guess I was just so pumped to be going to Berlin that I didn't give the events themselves a second thought. Ben and I knew what time I'd be aiming for in each event and the splits per round, so I'd always be aware of whether I was on pace or if I was playing catch-up, and that seemed like enough. I wanted to go in stress-free and maximise my enjoyment of the experience as a whole. As a result (perhaps there's wisdom in the phrase 'ignorance is bliss'!), I was not nervous at all, just extremely excited. I had taken all the pressure off myself and even though the stadium would be rammed full of 3,500 fans, I felt no nerves. All I wanted was to get out there and start soaking it all in.

Two days out from the event, I dropped into a CrossFit gym in Berlin with John and Leon, just to do some light conditioning, nothing too serious. At that time, the 'floss' dance was doing the rounds on social media and we were mucking around practising it. I said to John that I was going to do that dance after every event. He didn't believe me as he thought I'd be too battered from the workouts but I was determined to do it because I thought it would be funny and I'm always happiest when I'm making other people smile.

On the first day of the competition, the first event was three kilometres on the rower, three hundred double-unders – which is skipping but spinning the rope around twice per jump – and then three miles on an Air Runner treadmill. It was my first time on an Air Runner and if you're wondering how it's different to a normal treadmill, it's that there is no motor – the only thing that powers the belt around is your own effort and I was blowing hard. Halfway through the run, the Katy Perry song that started the floss dance came on over the PA system in the stadium; my family and friends were in my eyeline so I screamed over to John that this was the song and then did the dance while I was running. They all looked shocked and were waving at me to stop and shouting that I should concentrate but I was being myself and enjoying my first time on the Regionals stage. When I got off the Air Runner and crossed the finish line I flossed again and the whole crowd cheered. I paused for a moment and thought to myself that *this* was what I had come for.

CrossFit is renowned for its 'benchmark workouts' – sessions that let you gauge your strengths and weaknesses and chart improvement whenever you repeat them. Many of them had been given girls' names. Which, despite being odd, was not something I thought much about at the time, though it would later come to seem troubling. The second event at Regionals that year was called Linda. I definitely should have practised Linda.

The workout consists of 135kg deadlifts, 90kg bench presses and 65kg squat cleans, which you perform in a descending ladder from ten down to one. So, you do ten deadlifts, ten bench presses and then ten squat cleans. Then you go back and do nine of each movement, then eight, then seven and so on, until you finish with a round of a single rep of all three moves. My raw strength has always been really good, even back in the day when Harmeet saw me shoulder pressing 100 kg in the corner at Be Fitter Gym, so, despite not practising or working out any kind of strategy, I thought I was going to crush that event.

I started *very* hard on the round of ten, going full speed and not dropping the bar once on the squat cleans. In my head, I was going to maintain that pace all the way through; when the stadium MC announced that I was in the lead, I was even more determined to smash it. But then, in the round of seven, I got to the bench press and realised that I was totally exhausted. I had gone out far too hot and had paced it completely wrong. People who had gone at a more measured pace in the first long rounds started to overtake me and then accelerate as the rounds became shorter. I just died off even more as it went on.

I came across the finish line fourth in my heat and, even though I was knackered, broke out my floss dance with a huge smile on my face. My friends and I were cracking up laughing about how badly I paced it as they had never seen me die off during a workout like that but I wasn't bothered. Nothing could rock my ambition to seize the moment and I was already in love with being out on the competition floor at that level, performing the sport I was so deeply passionate about in front of thousands of fans in the building and thousands more who were watching the live stream from their homes. It felt like I belonged on that stage, that I was meant to be there. In the warm-up area and during the events themselves, I couldn't stop smiling.

Just after that workout, CrossFit posted a video of my

finish-line dancing on social media and my support in the stadium and online went through the roof. Everyone was going mental for it and I think I gained 7,000 followers on Instagram overnight. I think how much I was genuinely enjoying myself, how laid back I was compared to some of the other, super-intense competitors really resonated with people.

When you're chasing down a goal you have to really relish the achievements and victories along the way. It doesn't mean that you aren't serious about the bigger picture. My flossing and the happiness streaming out of me on that first day in Berlin, or when I was laughing after struggling through an event that I should have excelled at, in no way meant that I was not committed to getting to the CrossFit Games.

Yes, you should be constantly working towards your goals. But if your dream is big enough and there are countless steps to take over many years, you need to savour each win as you move through the process. If you don't, you might not last the whole course. You can only hit so many hurdles before it becomes disheartening, even if you are deeply passionate about what you're doing. Committing to those moments of enjoyment is an indelible reminder of why you're striving so hard for something. We all need to celebrate when we can.

When we got back to our hotel after the end of the first day of competition, John, Leon and I sat in my room chatting and laughing for so long that, before we knew it, it was way past midnight. When I realised the time I said, 'Lads! I've got to be back at the stadium in a few hours!' It wasn't the best

PICK A TIME

It can help to do your journaling at the same time every day. It can get you into the rhythm of the exercise and will make stopping for a few minutes easier. If you're taking photos then find a time at the end of the day to review the day's images.

START OFF SMALL

Don't be put off by the idea that you have to make grand, sweeping gestures. You are far better off beginning with the smallest things you can think of. Maybe you enjoyed the cup of coffee you had before starting your day. Or that the sun was out on your way to work. Start from there and build up if you feel up to it.

A huge part of CrossFit is being able to handle any form of physical challenge. In the Open, all the workouts have to be accessible to everyone and, as such, they all use equipment that every CrossFit gym should have. At Regionals, though, all the kit is provided on site, so HQ has the opportunity to surprise the athletes with what they refer to as the 'unknown and unknowable'. Waiting for me at the stadium that morning, after kicking around with my mates until the early hours, was a brand-new movement never seen before in competition.

There were rounds of two more classic moves – muscle-ups at one end of the floor, which start as a pull-up but you launch yourself right up and over the bar, and one-legged 'pistol' squats at the other, divided by two ramps that you had to walk over on your hands – up, over and down in between each movement. Handstand walks are a staple of CrossFit and almost always feature in live comps. I was OK at handstand walks but at six foot and 100kg, gymnastic moves were something that I was still working on improving to match my strength and fitness. But the ramps were new.

You didn't get to practise or even touch the ramps in the warm-up area but a few days before the competition we constructed one out of weight plates and whiteboards, so I could at least give it a go. I couldn't do it. I didn't manage to get up one side and down the other a single time. The whole workout wasn't great for me as pistol squats – a relatively simple CrossFit movement where you squat with one leg and hold the other in the air without touching the ground before swapping sides – were terrible for my ankles, which had continued to be an issue even after I stopped playing rugby. But I'd just thought I'd have to go out on the day and see what happened. Worrying about it all wasn't going to help, after all.

Just before the event started, I was chatting to another athlete from the UK called Will Kane, who's a friend of mine now, though back then we didn't really know each other. We were talking about the workout on the start line. I asked him if he was going to walk or jog back to the rings after each set of pistol squats and he looked at me like I was mad, 'No, mate. You've got to handstand walk back as well!' I just stood on the start line for a few seconds, coming to terms with the realisation that I didn't even know the workout properly and I had to attempt the ramp twice each round. Then the buzzer went off and we all kicked up onto our hands and started walking.

I got over and down the obstacle on the first try. I could hear all my supporters going nuts and the whole crowd seemed to swell in support. I was buzzing. I looked over to John and screamed, 'John, I did it!' He looked at me wide-eyed, waved me on and yelled back that I still had the whole workout to go and to get on with it. I carried on and managed the ramp again on the way back. I got through a few rounds but then my handstand walking started to break down as I got tired and I kept falling and having to go back and kick up again.

I tied for thirty-fourth out of the field of 40 and it was my worst finish of the whole competition. There was a time limit of 13 minutes and when the klaxon went, I did my dance and walked off the floor waving to my fans and supporters. A lot of athletes would have been really annoyed in that situation and been upset by their performance but I didn't feel any shame in my showing whatsoever. For me, getting over that ramp once was such a win and everything after that was a bonus, so it didn't matter to me what my placement was because I had exceeded my own expectations and performed better than I had thought I was able to. In the warm-up area

I had tried it 20 times and couldn't do it, so all my supporters were high-fiving me and telling me how well I had done. To look at it, you'd think I'd finished near the top in that workout! According to the leader board, obviously I did not. But through the lens of my mindset, I *had* won that morning.

By the time we got to the last event on the Sunday afternoon, my body was in pieces. I was sore and more exhausted than I'd ever felt doing CrossFit. Six highly competitive workouts over three days was the first time I'd experienced not only that sort of workload but also the intensity. Every event was an absolute max effort. But despite not being up there in the final heat contending for a top five spot and a ticket to the Games, I was getting huge amounts of support and kept getting stopped for pictures. People were asking me to sign their T-shirts and hats and that was when I started to realise that there was a genuine opportunity for this to be my career, as well as my sport – that people and brands would want to be associated with my name.

I know that all came from how much I committed to making those three days as much fun as I possibly could. I finished the weekend in twenty-eighth, a full 23 places away from the qualification line of fifth or better. You could say that in terms of my overall dream of going to the Crossfit Games, that weekend was not a success. But in truth, it's the perfect example of setting a big goal yet understanding that you've got smaller targets to hit along the way and being realistic with yourself about where you are.

When you hit those waypoints, every time you climb a rung on the ladder, you have to rejoice in those moments. You should celebrate each win, even the smallest ones. If you don't, the process will never be truly enjoyable. If you ignore the value in improvement and how it is cast-iron evidence of your dedication and effort, trying to achieve your goals will cease to be fun. You will lose the passion you had to walk your path; it will become nothing but a constant grind. Even a person with extreme motivation and rock solid self-belief will get worn down by grinding day-in and day-out for months and years on end. In fitness or business, at home or at work, committing to every moment of your development as you move towards your goal is something worth celebrating. It's the only way you'll get there.

CUT OUT THE NOISE

It is human nature for the mind to wander but becoming distracted from what you're actually doing can have a greater impact than simply slowing down your progress. In fact, being more present in the moment on a regular basis can make you happier and more motivated.

Psychologists at Harvard University collated information on the daily actions, thoughts and feelings of over 2,000 volunteers to discover how often they were fully concentrating on their tasks and what made them happiest. The conclusion was that thinking about the past or daydreaming about the future made people more miserable.

Being more present does not mean you have to meditate. Next time you go out for a walk or on the commute to work, leave your headphones behind and focus on everything around you instead. By being aware of the rhythm of your feet striking the ground or noticing the interesting roof of a building you pass every day but have never seen before, you can unlock the boost in happiness of being in the moment.

I understood what sort of athlete I was in 2018. I knew I wasn't good enough to qualify for the Games then. I didn't let that get me down because I believed that one day I would be ready to make that jump. If you're looking for a promotion or a new job but you know that you're not ready yet, there is no point getting stressed about it. If you think you'll be in a position to apply in a year, commit to getting the best out of yourself and enjoying your work as much as you can. Being annoyed every month that you still haven't got anywhere will only ruin your chances of moving up.

I was acutely aware that I wasn't going to be contending for a top five spot at Regionals in 2018. But by going into that weekend with a positive attitude I took away some lessons that would set me up for success in the years to come. I learned that I would never fail to be prepared for a workout ever again and I discovered that I deal well with pressure and thrive in the atmosphere of higher-level competitions. I worked out that I absorbed huge amounts of positive energy being in front of the crowd from people cheering and celebrating. And perhaps most importantly, I found out that I liked the sort of person I was becoming as an athlete.

When I got home and came down from the buzz of Berlin, all the workouts and the intensity of the experience caught up with me and it had a massive impact on my body. I was sore for days and days afterwards and then I got tonsillitis, so I was ill for about a month. It gave me time to take stock, though, and assess where I was in my grander plan.

The 2018 Eurpean Regional was a huge confidence booster. That I could be relaxed and enjoy myself that much, that I could dance on the finish line and shout over to my friends in the crowd mid-workout and *still* finish in the middle of the pack. So I worked out the steps I needed to take next. I would focus more on my nutrition to make sure I was always primed to perform every day. I was going to work even less so I could train more and recover better.

Being around the top-level guys in Europe gave me a clear roadmap to how I should approach competitions as a professional athlete. When I was walking around the arena in Berlin, I was shocked that all these people had their own coaches and always had tubs of their own pre-prepared food with them. I remember thinking that there was no messing around with these guys, while I was strolling around backstage on my own and begging my friends to go out into the city to find me something vaguely good to eat in between events. If I wanted to get to the pinnacle of CrossFit, I needed to take things more seriously and ensure every aspect of my training and competing was taken care of.

But I was going to have some fun in the process.

YOUR SWOS PROGRAMME

The first stage of being able to overcome hurdles in any area of your life is to make the most of every win, no matter how big or small. Enjoying yourself as much as you're able to is not fooling yourself – you should see living and savouring the moment as a way of topping up your fuel tank of motivation. Each time you improve, even slightly, instantly provides positive physical and mental feedback, which then feeds your desire to reach the next level, whatever it may be.

We're going to begin with the notes you've been making so far at the back of the book or in your phone or notebook. Go back over what you wrote in the first section of the book and select a smaller aspect of your overall goal that you can build up to over time. Then work out how you can chip away to reach the first milestone. You'll find space to write your thoughts down on page 233.

If your ambition is to learn to play the guitar, say, pick a simple song that you think you can get the hang of with a bit of practice, then commit to spending 20 minutes a day working on it.

Or use a simple workout movement as an example – the push-up. You're going to do five push-ups every minute for 10 minutes. You can do them on your knees or with your hands on a surface like a step or a chair, or regular push-ups if you can do them. Start a stopwatch, do five reps and then rest for the remainder of the minute. Then, when the second minute rolls around, do another five and then rest. Continue for ten minutes and, before you know it, you will have done 50 push-ups.

The week after, add an extra push-up per minute for a total of 60 reps. The week after, see if you can do seven per minute. You're only adding a single rep at a time but it adds up to significant progress that you can and should enjoy. If you can get up to ten push-ups per minute and reach 100 in total that is a genuine milestone.

Or when, after a week of practice, you can play that song perfectly, that is a reason to celebrate. So celebrate!

In the next chapter, we will be looking at how to deal with failure and turn it to your advantage. We have to enjoy ourselves at every available opportunity, otherwise, when things do get tough, we won't have the reserves of willpower to stick it out.

CHAPTER FIVE

FIND STRENGTH IN WEAKNESS

We all have stuff we're good at and some things we could do better. If we're honest, there are often aspects that we are really bad at. You might be performing well in your career but not great with money, for example. Or you're a good friend that has a habit of forgetting birthdays. Those nuances are OK and it's what makes you a person. Even the most successful of people have areas in their life that aren't as optimal as others.

What successful people tend to do, however, is evaluate where they can improve and then take that as an opportunity to level up. They view weaknesses as the ground most fertile for fresh growth, where they can build new strength to become a more rounded person, employee, parent or athlete. They seek to balance out their abilities so that their natural skills aren't limited by a glaring inability.

After a break from training to get my health and body

back together, I was raring to get back into the gym and start ironing out my own imbalances and improving my fitness for what I was sure was going to be my best season yet. I was riding the wave of confidence that competing at Regionals gives you; the feeling of being one of the best in Europe and good enough to compete at that level fed into every single rep of all my workouts that year. Most of all, knowing that I had not taken myself too seriously and I had absolutely loved the experience told me that I was ready.

Going into the 2019 CrossFit season, I had planned out the steps I needed to take. I was good enough now not to stress about the Open so much as I knew I could make the top 40 in the region. That meant I would schedule my training in order to be in peak physical condition at Regionals. I now understood the quality of athlete I'd have to be in order to finish in the top five and knew that if I made the right adjustments, in competition as well as training, I could do it. I felt like I knew exactly what I was dealing with.

Then CrossFit HQ announced they were going to change the sport. The season that we as athletes had all worked towards for years was going to operate completely differently and Regionals were not part of that plan. Instead of progressing from the Open to Regionals and then to the Games, there would now be a more convoluted system of qualification. The top 20 athletes in the world on the Open leader board would automatically go straight through to the Games. Instead of Regionals, there would be 16 officially sanctioned events, quickly dubbed Sanctionals, which would each offer Games invites to their overall winners. Finally, and most dramatically, any country with at least one properly affiliated CrossFit gym would crown their man and woman with the top Open results as their national champion, all of whom would get a direct invite to the CrossFit Games.

The impact on us as athletes was seismic. I think if there's a change in any sport, your initial reaction is to hate it. We like to know what we're dealing with but there was no warning and it just seemed like an ultimatum from CrossFit's CEO and owner at the time, Greg Glassman. As more details emerged, it was evident that he was indeed intending to change everything. I was actually in favour of globalising the sport but I took issue with the structure that had been put in place and was especially put out by how harshly it had been dropped on the community.

You can always find some positives in even the worst situations, though. As they announced the Sanctionals they included all the top-flight competitions around the world, which meant that athletes would be able to travel around the world, from Dubai to Miami via Iceland and Minnesota with the chance to go up against the top people to compete for an invite to the Games and earn prize money in the process. It was an opportunity to get outside of my European bubble and compete with the big names of the sport.

The biggest impact on me, though, I quickly realised, was that I stood a genuine chance of coming first in the UK in the Open and immediately punching my ticket. I wouldn't have the stress of a full-on weekend at Regionals where one bad workout could leave you outside the top five. I wouldn't even have to worry about winning a Sanctional. If I was first in the UK in the Open then I could just focus on being the strongest and fittest I had *ever* been by the time I got on the plane to the CrossFit Games. I was, suddenly, only one step away from that dream.

I immediately overhauled my season-long training pro-gramme to plant my whole focus on the Open, which was now going to be held in the coming autumn, rather than spring the following year as before. I wanted to give everything I had for those five Open workouts and get myself straight through to the Games. Best of all, I could get it done early.

ACCEPT WEAKNESS

Weakness is an inevitability of life and we all have chinks in our armour. But finding a hole in your game, whether that's in your professional skillset, on the sports field or dealing with the day-to-day at home, is not some-thing to shy away from. Weaknesses will always come around and that will never change. As with external forces, be that an unexpected bill, or something more serious such as a family member falling ill, our reac-tion is the only way to redefine the situation.

There are some simple tools to reframe and make our response more positive. Next time you receive less-than-ideal news, try the following.

TAKE A BREATH

And sit down for a minute. When negative news hits, it has the double-whammy effect of raising our heart rate and unmooring us psychologically. Sitting down and taking a few deep breaths both slows your BPM and puts you physically in one place, giving your mind the time it needs to regain some composure.

SPEAK TO SOMEONE

Very few of us can handle disappointment on our own. As you process the news, try to move straight into thinking about who would be best to talk to. Perhaps it's as simple as calling a friend to vent about the issue. For something more serious, you might need to contact someone who can offer professional help, like a doctor or lawyer.

MAKE A PLAN

It's hard to launch into planning mode immediately. But even figuring out a general idea of the steps you

can take to proceed can flip your mindset into a positive mode. Not all things can be handled with action
– sometimes comprehending and processing it emo-
tionally is a plan in and of itself. If you can accept that
you're already on your way to new-found strength.

I took on the first workout of the 2019 CrossFit Open at
a UK competition called Strength in Depth. The announce-
ment from HQ that overhauled the season was so sudden that
I had already agreed to take part by then. In fact, because
the Open had been brought forward by over three months,
the Strength in Depth organisers had to keep the first slot on
Friday clear in order that all the athletes could do the Open
workout as an event that would also count towards their final
score for the competition. I was fully aware that a full two
days of competition could leave me sore for a good week
afterwards when I wanted to be in top condition, but I had
established in Berlin the year before that I loved performing
and this was a huge UK event. I wanted to throw down in
front of a home crowd.

We had, of course, planned to do all the Open workouts
at CrossFit BFG, where I would have three or four of my
team around me with whom I could discuss strategies before
each attempt. There would be people with stopwatches tim-
ing my splits to make sure I wasn't going out too hard. Ben
would have our full strategy mapped out on the whiteboard

and sometimes even a plan B on a separate board in case we wanted to change tactics mid-workout. The Open events were going to be a massive team effort.

But at Strength in Depth, the atmosphere and crowd meant I just went as hard as I could. We had 15 minutes to get through as many rounds as possible of rowing for 19 calories followed by 19 wall balls – throwing a 9kg medicine ball to a 10-foot target directly above you. I almost pulled the rowing machine to bits on the first few rounds and when I looked at the clock and saw that I was only seven minutes in, I thought that I had really screwed up. You can't help but race the other athletes, so my game plan went straight out the window. I still got a decent enough score. Not amazing, but it was OK considering the situation. Unfortunately, I had to withdraw from the rest of the competition because I had a knee injury which was giving me a bit of an issue and I needed to make sure I was in shape for the rest of the Open.

On the Monday, back at CrossFit BFG, I told my crew that I had to repeat the workout. My legs were pretty blown from the weekend but Ben had worked out the splits I had to hit on the whiteboard and was shouting out if I was just under or over as I moved through round after round of rowing and wall balls. Some of our members, the coaches and Sam were screaming and constantly pushing me on. It was so much easier than at the competition purely because I paced it so well. I beat my previous score by 20–30 reps.

Once all the scores had been registered on the Monday,

I was fourth in the UK. It wasn't a perfect start but it was a good one all the same. The second workout was released and the movements were good for me, with rounds of toes-to-bar, double-unders and cleans with an increasingly heavy barbell. Toes-to-bar – where you hang from the bar and bring your toes up to touch the pull-up bar – are one of the less technical gymnastic movements and, with my natural strength, it's always to my advantage whenever a heavy barbell is involved.

As a result, I won that workout convincingly; in fact, I was the only man in the UK to finish all 430 reps before the 20-minute time limit. With a fourth and first place in the two events so far, I was right where I needed to be, so it felt like it was all going to plan.

Then the third workout of 2019 came along and it was, without a doubt, the biggest upset of my career so far. It read as follows:

200-foot dumbbell overhead lunge
50 dumbbell box step-ups
50 strict handstand push-ups
200-foot handstand walk

As I've mentioned before, I'm six foot tall and weigh 100kg, so gymnastic movements that require you to move your bodyweight with power, skill and precision had always been something I struggled with. Lighter people have less to move, so tend to be more suited to things like muscle-ups or handstand walking. Those on the shorter end have a biome-chanical advantage, as shorter limbs have less far to travel and therefore take less effort.

I had been practising kipping handstand press-ups, when you bend your legs and then shoot them upwards as you press to use momentum to make things easier on your shoulders, as it's the most efficient way to do multiple reps. Having to perform them 'strict' meant no kipping was allowed and you had to keep your legs locked out at all times. I hadn't been doing any in training because it had never come up in the Open before.

I knew I wasn't going to place near the top of the UK leader board on that workout, so I just needed to avoid an absolute disaster. As long as I did all right and didn't totally bomb, I was confident that I could still win and qualify as national champion. I went into the gym and watched some of the members do the event and thought it didn't look too bad. My training partners turned up that evening as usual to do the workout with me. We warmed up, set the timer for ten minutes and got down to it.

You can only do the walking lunges and box step-ups so fast, so we were all pretty much level when we kicked up on the wall for the strict handstand press-ups. But after 15–20 reps, I totally redlined. I couldn't do more than one or two at a time and was having to rest longer and longer to try to shake out the burning sensation in my shoulders. Even the reps I was managing I had to *really* fight for.

My score was terrible. My team, who just train for fun, completed all the work within the time cap and they smashed the workout compared to me. I hadn't even made it to the handstand walk before the buzzer went off, I was struggling with the hand-stand press-ups so much. I couldn't afford to do that poorly if I wanted to make it to the Games but, strangely, I wasn't worried – I thought I'd just approached it the wrong way and my strategy wasn't right, so I decided I would just have another go at the workout and try to improve my score.

I came back to the gym on Saturday with a new plan. I felt like I had been overconfident with my strict handstand press-ups the day before and had done big sets linked together to start with, which must have burned out my shoulders. I had been doing sets of eights but I was going to pace it better this time and break them up into smaller sets of four or so. I told myself that I would smash it this time.

I did even *worse* that second time and that's when I started to feel like I was in a bit of trouble. I got to the wall at roughly the same point, so it wasn't the lunges or the box step-ups, I just couldn't do the strict handstand press-ups and my training partners kept beating me as my scores spiralled downwards. That afternoon, we tried out another strategy but only as a trial and not to complete the workout. It didn't look like it was going to work so I decided to take a complete rest day on Sunday and then have another run at it on Monday, as my shoulders and triceps were seriously aching by this point.

On Monday morning I attempted the workout for a fourth

time. It was my last shot and I was willing to try anything to make sure this event didn't ruin my overall placing. I'd been trying all night to figure out a better way to break down the work and had decided I was going to do all the handstand press-ups as single reps. I was going to kick up, do one rep, come back down, rest for a second and then kick back up again for another. Fifty single reps was the only thing left for me to try and all my crew were geeing me up, telling me, 'You've got it this time! Singles mean your shoulders won't burn out. Just go for it!' Nobody showed any doubt and I didn't allow anything else other than the workout to come into my mind, even though deep down I knew that I was going to struggle to improve as much as I needed to.

I did the lunges and the box step-ups and reached the wall at the same time as all my other attempts, then kicked up against the wall, performed one handstand press-up and then came back down, as planned. Ten single reps in, I suddenly admitted to myself that I just wasn't good enough. After 20 reps, I was way off the pace and I said to Harmeet, 'I think we should stop,' and we ended it there.

Everyone was saying 'well done' and all those things that you say to be nice but I just wanted to go home, chill and not talk to anyone. I had tried so many different ways to get around the handstand press-ups but I simply couldn't do them. When all the results were in, I ended up coming 168th in that workout and my goal disappeared out of reach in an instant, when it had been so close. People were messaging me, saying 'Come on, Zack. It's not over and anything can happen between now and the end of the Open.' But they knew as well as I did that I'd screwed my chances of winning.

I was very, very upset. I was annoyed at myself because it was my own fault – I hadn't been practising strict handstand press-ups and that was on me. I had a bit of a pity party for the rest of that day on Monday but as soon as we were into our normal training that week, I mentally turned the page. I wasn't going to win the Open now. But I wanted to prove how dominant I could be in the remaining events. I could have just gone through the motions for the last two workouts but I didn't quit when others might well have done. I ended up winning the fourth workout and finishing second in the final event.

The glaring weakness that had been exposed by the third workout in 2019 had cost me a spot at the CrossFit Games. But I was proud of the mental resilience I had shown by finishing the Open strong. The hyper-competitive part of me wanted to make sure that the athletes that were ranked above me knew that I had lost out because of one movement, not that they had beaten me. I had to prove to myself that I was good enough, had it not been for that awful workout.

Elliot Simmonds, who finished first and was crowned the UK national champion, texted me after all the results were finalised, saying, 'Great battle in the Open. Thank God you can't do handstand press-ups!' Elliot got the invite to the CrossFit Games. He hadn't won any of the workouts but he only finished worse than fourth once, and even then only came eleventh. I won two of the events, got second in one and fourth in another. But my worst score, that handstand press-up workout, was 168th.

WELCOME THE FEEDBACK

Failure of any kind is usually at least a little demoralising. To feel no disappointment when you don't live up the expectations you have for yourself, or that others have set upon you, is impossible in the moment. In fact, if you think back to your Start Where Others Stop programme at the end of Chapter Three, when you imagined how you would feel if you didn't achieve your goal, feeling disappointment was one of the key signifiers that your goal is one you are passionate about.

When the mental dust has settled, and you should grant yourself the time for this process to take its natural time, try to view missteps as valuable feedback and something you can use to improve. This comes down to asking better questions of yourself and avoiding falling back into negativity. The following are a good start:

1) What is the one thing I could learn from this situation?

---

2) How can I tweak my plan to avoid making this mistake again?

3) What is the one thing I will do differently the next time?

Don't rush with these. Some might occur to you immediately whereas others may require more thought over a number of days. It's important to answer them honestly, as it will help you move forward and turn a failure into future success. Good luck!

Two months later, I took part in my first Sanctional of the new season format. The CrossFit Lowlands Throwdown took place in the Netherlands at the end of May and it was a competition I felt I could win and secure a Games invite as a result. Finishing the Open so well had given me a huge mental boost and had helped put the disappointment of the handstand press-ups to bed, so I wanted to put in a good performance and keep moving forward.

The first group of workouts went well and I was in contention for the top spot but again I got tripped up by an event that really didn't suit me. In fact, if I had to pick a truly terrible combination for me, that workout would be close. It was 50, 40, 30, 20 and 10 reps of sit-ups on a piece of equipment called a GHD – an elevated stand into which you secure

in a number of different formats. The result was to put them in an EMOM, which stands for 'every minute on the minute', doing a few reps each time a new minute starts and then resting for the remainder. Sometimes I would do one rep every 30 seconds or I'd put handstand press-ups in the middle of a workout to get used to performing them under fatigue.

Repeating those formats and adding a rep each week was an easy way to chart my progression. I was fully committed to practising the movement every other day. I was relentless; my poor training partners would come into the gym and ask me what we were doing that day and they would all roll their eyes when I wrote handstand press-ups on the board again. But I didn't care. I was adamant that I would never get caught out on that move if it came up in competition. We all did a *lot* of handstand press-ups getting ready for the 2020 Open, which, unusually, that year was actually in October 2019 (they're normally in February). I'd later realise that this was yet another case of the season being chopped and changed around seemingly without any thought for the athletes.

For the first time since I was a child, I also decided to cut a bit of weight. I realised I could become as technically proficient at gymnastics as I wanted but if I lost three or four kilos it would massively boost my ability. I could be exactly the same in terms of skill and strength on handstand press-ups but being lighter would allow me to do extra reps. It doesn't sound like much but carrying four fewer kilos makes a palpable difference to your performance and you're instantly better.

FIND STRENGTH IN WEAKNESS

This is because to transform a weakness into a real strength, the most important thing is to go further than you have to. A lot of people do what they are told and then stop – they are content doing what is required of them but nothing more and, while they will improve, they will find it impossible to become really proficient at something that once was an obvious flaw. That mentality so obviously relates to your career. If you simply do what is asked of you, nobody will complain. You're doing your job, after all. If you do that extra bit, though, if you use your initiative to come up with a smarter system, or a better way of bringing in new business, your career progress is guaranteed to be enhanced.

Training my strict handstand press-ups three times a week was what I *had* to do as a professional athlete. But by going that bit further and going on a small weight cut before the start of the next Open, I had supercharged my improvement as I was both stronger and leaner. I had attacked my weakness on both fronts.

In that awful workout that lost me the national championship earlier that year, it had taken me five-and-a-half minutes to do the 50 handstand press-ups on my best attempt. After training them methodically and dropping down to 96kg, I had brought that down to two minutes and twenty seconds, which means I had more than doubled my strength and proficiency at the movement. Heading into my second Open of the year, that turnaround gave my confidence and self-belief a little top up at the perfect time.

The first workout released was ten rounds of eight barbell snatches and ten burpees jumping over the bar. I was actually in Tenerife with John and Leon hosting a fitness retreat on the first Friday, so we did it out there in the heat. The snatches – taking the bar from the ground to overhead in one movement – were light at only 43kg, so it was going to be a raw test of capacity: who could set a fast but sustainable pace and hang on through all 180 total reps. As soon as I started moving, I felt the benefit of being that little bit lighter. It felt good.

I flew back with plenty of time to get the plane ride out of my system and repeat the workout on the Monday. With the benefit of the tester I'd done while away, I paced it perfectly and won the workout on the UK leader board. It couldn't have gone better and I was the only man in the UK to finish the workout in under nine minutes.

The national championship was a three-horse race for the 2020 season. Elliot and I had been joined by David Shorunke and we were all jostling for position. After two weeks, I was sitting in third behind Elliot and David and then the third workout was released. It contained no fewer than 45 handstand push-ups and 150 feet of handstand walking. It wasn't the same as the event that had blown my chances earlier in the year but it was close enough! The exact details were:

21 deadlifts, 115kg
21 handstand push-ups
15 deadlifts, 115kg

15 handstand push-ups
9 deadlifts, 115kg
9 handstand push-ups
21 deadlifts, 143kg
50ft handstand walk
15 deadlifts, 143kg
50ft handstand walk
9 deadlifts, 143kg
50ft handstand walk
Time cap: 9 minutes

Everyone knew that handstand push-ups had been a huge weakness of mine and Elliot even said in a podcast after the Open was over that he had thought that was me out of the running when the workout was announced. But I knew how much work I'd put in to eradicate that hole in my game and I was naturally good at deadlifts, so I didn't just want to do better than the year before. My aim wasn't only to avoid totally tanking – I wanted to own this workout. I wanted to crush it.

We set up everything perfectly back home at CrossFit BFG on the Friday night. We had a massive crowd there, as everyone knew that this was my moment to make a real statement and they all wanted to give me whatever help they could. The team and I were happy with the strategy and all that was left to do was to go for it.

I smashed the deadlifts and the handstand push-ups went better than anyone expected, then I flew through the handstand walks and finished in 7 minutes and 36 seconds. As it's an online competition, you have no idea how your score stacks up but I was extremely happy with how it went. I knew that Elliot and David would be looking at the movements and thinking that I wasn't even going to finish before the time cap, so I was pumped about my performance. Now I just had to wait and see how the other two had got on.

The next day I was *extremely* sore. The combination of bracing my whole body to stay stable on all the deadlifts and then squeezing my core as tight as possible on the handstand movements made it very taxing on the body. Come the Monday, my body was still fatigued and I came into the gym to repeat the workout and try and improve my score. While I was warming up at about 5 p.m. I felt heavy and sluggish and by 7 p.m. I still hadn't done the event. I said to the team that I was going to wait and see what scores came in from the other two. If I had to do it again to beat them, I would. Shorunke's time came in and he was way off my pace, finishing a full minute behind me. Then, finally, Elliot's popped up on the leader board. He was 20 seconds slower than me.

To come first in the UK when everyone from my direct competitors to CrossFit analysts expected me to struggle was a massive achievement and it was far and away the proudest moment of my career so far. I had turned a weakness, something that had stopped me from reaching my goals, into a strength. I was never going to be the best in the world at handstand press-ups, yet all that time practising in the gym gave me the leg-up I needed to make it over the wall. There were two workouts to go but I couldn't help but feel the momentum was with me.

RETHINKING FAILURE

The idea that you can learn from failure is not just a slogan. A study published in the journal *Frontiers in Psychology* found that reacting to setbacks with a positive growth mindset made the biggest difference to achieving goals rather than falling short.

The researchers conducted interviews on athletes from football, rowing, skiing and combat sports to establish any difference in personality traits between elite athletes and those who never quite made it to the top. They focused specifically on their career trajectory, the obstacles they had faced and how they reacted to those challenges.

The researchers concluded that the elite show a commitment to their goals that the near-elite did not. More crucially, they found that following a failure, the high performers showed a desire to return stronger than ever as soon as possible, whereas their less successful colleagues tended to lose their enthusiasm.

There was very little variation in how many challenges all of the people studied faced – the defining factor is how you react to those failures. Think back now to your last failure and list as many things you learned from the experiences as possible. Start small and work your way up to the bigger picture. Congratulations – you're already turning a weakness into a strength. Learning from your mistakes and seeing failure as a positive force is what can make you a champion of your field.

That confidence and my mindset was truly tested again the following week. Elliot and I were tied for first at the top of the leader board but the fourth workout contained movements that were physically very hard for me with my history of injuries. Pistol squats were in there – the same exercise that had cost me at the Lowlands Throwdown and would always cause my knee to flare up. Box jumps featured, too, which with my ankles were a real problem – I can't jump down and bounce straight into the next rep like most people, so I always had to take them slowly.

Among all the pistols and box jumps, were barbell clean and jerks, so that was good for me. The repetitions decreased each round but the weight went up and it was quite heavy towards the end of the workout, though it didn't get heavy enough for me to feel like Elliot had no chance of lifting it. I was going to have to grind and fight *again*. I had been so confident I was going to win the Open but on the Friday morning I was lying in bed and the doubt was starting to seep in – I couldn't believe the two movements I couldn't physically improve upon might take my dream away.

When I walked into the gym, I could see in their faces that they thought it was already over for me. Everyone looked really sad because they all knew that pistols mangled my knees and ankles and that I couldn't go fast on box jumps. They were right to be concerned but seeing how much it was worrying my whole team, my family and friends, helped me mentally flip a switch. I was going to attack this workout positively and tactically and I wasn't going to let that Games invite get snatched away from me.

So I stepped up and stepped down from the box on every rep and took the pistol squats at a steady pace to make sure I did each one perfectly and didn't tweak my knee or crush my ankles. Being four kilograms lighter really helped again as I felt far less pressure going through my joints on the squats. Then I went as hard as I could on the barbell to make up as much time as possible between each set of the bodyweight movements.

I was happy with my time but we decided to leave it a couple of days to let my ankles and knees recover and then repeat the workout on the Monday to try to better my score. As ever, we had a board with the splits I needed to hit in order to get faster. We also had a strategy in place to ensure I was pushing it fast on the barbell but not so fast that I ended up having to rest too long towards the end. I beat my first attempt and finished with a time of 16 minutes and 59 seconds. We celebrated like mad because we all knew that I had done the absolute best that I could in an event that was not set up for me to excel.

I came second in the UK on that workout, which was a massive achievement. I could have rolled over and admitted defeat or given myself the excuse that the injuries I'd had when I was younger held me back and it couldn't be helped. My team and I pulled together and found a way to make it work when we really had to.

BUILD THE RIGHT TEAM

We all know that teams can be very effective but some teams work better than others. And just because you are working with other people, it doesn't mean that you are functioning well as a team. Genuine teamwork means that you are collaborating, communicating and that you all share a common purpose. Just because you have set yourself an individual goal, it doesn't mean that others don't share that ambition or aren't invested in your vision.

Building a team of any size – and just one other person counts – can provide a huge boost to your progress. Use this quick checklist to assess your team, or when constructing a new one:

David Shorunke won that week but, crucially, Elliot was further behind, finishing fourth, so the barbell had slowed him down after all. That left me in first and gave me a two-point buffer over Elliot in second place. There was just one workout between me and the realisation of a goal that I'd set myself six years earlier. The movements that could have tripped me up were out of the way and I'd made it over or around them and exceeded my potential. Anything that came up in week five was going to be a strength of mine.

On the face of it, the final workout was great for me. It was 40 ring muscle-ups, rowing until the read-out showed 80 calories and 120 wall balls, which are all exercises that suit me and my build. My gymnastics was the best it had ever been and rowing and wall balls are two of the few movements in CrossFit where being heavier and taller are a direct advantage. Each pull on the rowing machine you make is a bit longer and stronger and you don't have to throw the ball as far because you're closer to the target compared to an athlete who's five-foot-eight, for example.

There was a catch, though. In CrossFit competitions of any sort, there almost always is. For the first time ever that last week, it was entirely up to you as to how you partitioned the movements. You could split them up into 10 even rounds of 4 muscle-ups, 8 calories on the rower and 12 wall balls, if you liked, or do all the reps of one movement at a time – it was all down to what was best for you.

It was a neat twist but it resulted in all of us competitors repeating that workout over and over again, tweaking our strategies endlessly to maximise that vital last score. I was happy with my first effort on the Friday but knew I had to keep trying different ways of breaking up the reps to find the fastest method. The stress was unbearable and my crew and I were spending hours and hours every day trying to devise the optimal game plan. We did it again on the Saturday with a completely new strategy but it didn't work nearly as well. I rested on Sunday so I could make a final attempt on Monday before we needed to submit my time. I couldn't bear to imagine my goal slipping through my fingers again.

We decided to do ten fast rounds of the ring muscle-ups and wall balls and leave the row to the end and just go for it. I'll never forget being on that rower. There were over 40 people crowded around me cheering with every pull and the class that was going on at the time stopped and added to the screaming surge of supporters. When I reached 50 calories I was blowing hard but Ben told me that I was not on track to beat my time. I was not going to nearly kill myself without improving my score, so I ignored the pain and pulled even harder as the crowd went nuts. The atmosphere was insane. The last 10 calories were a complete blur and when I got to 80 I collapsed off the rower and just lay there as everyone mobbed me. I had set a new best time of 10 minutes and 33 seconds.

It was a nervous few hours after that, as I was holding on for Elliot to register his score before I put mine in and I was

YOUR SWOS PROGRAMME

As people, we tend to be very specific about our strengths. We say things like, 'I'm a great runner over short distances.' But when we feel like we are weak at something, then we almost always speak in general terms, so it becomes 'running just isn't for me'. But if you apply the same specificity to your perceived inabilities as you do to your merits, you can discover where your strengths really are and how to play to them.

Use the template on page 235 or take a piece of paper and draw three columns, headed 'Weaknesses', 'Strengths' and 'Changes'. In the first column, write down what you see as your weak points. They can be big or small, the process is the same. In the second column, think about where you are strong in the same area. Then, in the third column, write down what you can do to emphasise column two over column one. Here are some examples to give you the idea.

WEAKNESSES

I'm a bad writer and struggle with work emails

I never seem to have time to get everything done

I just can't lose any weight, even though I train daily

STRENGTHS

I'm great at talking and connecting with people

When I can concentrate I complete tasks perfectly

I am really strong and can lift much heavier than most

CHANGES

Use more phone and video calls when I'm at work

Focus on the one thing that will have the biggest impact

Work on building strength, rather than losing weight

You can apply this same device to any area in your life that you perceive to be weaker than others. As with the previous evaluation exercises we've covered in the Start Where Others Stop programme, it helps to begin as small as possible, so try to fight your natural urge to generalise. It's much easier to get to grips with 'I always hit the snooze button four or five times in the morning' than 'I'm a lazy person'.

With a bit of practice, you'll find you improve quite quickly and the better you're able to understand your weaknesses as an opportunity to find your strengths. In the next chapter, we'll be taking this one step further by learning how to use major setbacks as a springboard for success.

CHAPTER 6

USE SETBACKS AS LAUNCH PADS

Qualifying for the CrossFit Games had been my ultimate goal since 2013. By the time the 2020 event in Madison, Wisconsin, rolled round it would have been a seven-year journey to get there. All the mad training sessions that I squeezed in around pulling ten-hour days at our commercial gym and the local competitions where I had no idea what I was doing. The hundreds of workouts with Harmeet and hundreds more once I transferred into being a full-time athlete and started programming for myself. The highs of our week in Berlin and the lows of losing the national champion spot because of one workout. All the steps I had put in place and each milestone I passed were integral to getting me to the Games. It was the moment that I had been waiting for and one that, true to my mindset, I wanted to celebrate.

On that night when we were refreshing the leader board and waiting for Elliot's time to come in, I was sitting on the sofa at home with Sam, I was exhausted. My whole life had been consumed by the workouts over the last five weeks and, as much as it takes a huge physical toll, I was mentally burned out from constantly thinking about all the various rep schemes and strategies I could use to better each and every score. When all the scores were in and I was still on top, we got stuck into some food. Because I'd been on such a tight diet to trim down to 96kg, we ate a load of Maltesers, sticky toffee pudding and donuts. It was just like treat nights with Mum all those years ago.

But in the coming days, I didn't feel like I'd really won. Although I was in first position on the leader board, there were still countless workout videos that needed to be verified by CrossFit HQ, so even though I had done the hard part, I wouldn't let myself fully celebrate. I couldn't, not while there was still a chance that I might have some reps deducted or one of my times was adjusted. It had been such a tight race between Elliot, David and me that if I lost two reps in one workout, or had a few seconds added to another, then that would have been that.

I just wasn't myself. I hadn't been for almost two months. I wasn't upset or annoyed but nor was I over the moon. Despite the fact I had achieved my goal of winning the UK Open, I couldn't focus on anything because, in the back of my head, I was always waiting for that validation. Sam would be talking to me and, after a few minutes, I'd suddenly snap out of my day-dream and realise that I hadn't heard a word she was saying.

If you push that hard for something, stay the course for so long and find the result isn't what you expected, it's impossible not to feel deflated. Sometimes, our goals don't quite turn out as we dreamed. My plan of opening a chain of Be Fitter gyms certainly wasn't at all how I imagined, for example, but stumbling blocks of any sort don't have to halt your progress. In fact, even the biggest blow can set you up for even greater success. Setbacks, when approached with the Start Where Others Stop mindset, can be the most powerful launch pads in any area of your life.

With the Coronavirus pandemic that started sweeping the globe so tragically in early 2020, you might not be shocked to learn that I did not go to the CrossFit Games. What might surprise you is that I transformed it into the best thing that could have happened to me.

Of course, in autumn 2019, we had no idea what was lurking round the corner. After taking that first weekend off to chill with Sam, I decided that I was going to carry on like everything was normal. I woke up on the Monday morning threw on my kit and headed to the gym like I always do. The usual crowd was there and we started warming up. But before we had even started working out, I just didn't feel up for it, so I said goodbye and went home. The lads at the gym didn't know what to say, as they'd never seen me like that before – I *always* trained, even when I wasn't totally up for it. Normally, if I felt a bit unmotivated and complained about things, one of my crew would tell me to shut up, remind me that I was a professional athlete and I'd admit they were right, then crack on. During those first weeks after winning the Open, though, I came into train then promptly turned around and left probably seven or eight times. Sometimes I didn't even do the warm-up before jumping back in my car.

It was the first time I had ever experienced feeling like that. The year before, when I came down with tonsilitis, there was an obvious reason why I felt drained but after that Open I wasn't ill or injured and I just couldn't understand what was happening. I told myself, 'Come on, tomorrow will be better,' but then the next day would come along and it would not be better, so I'd just keep trying to talk myself into it over and over again.

It was only after speaking to a few people that I understood that I had probably had the most stressful five weeks of my life. It had been a full-speed rollercoaster of emotions going up and down every day for over a month and I hadn't given myself any real time to chill out mentally. I learned a lot from that feeling. Now, after a big competition, I will always give myself three weeks off from training to completely chill out. A full month, even. I need that time to give my body a chance to recover. More importantly, after the pressure of performing at my maximum level for weeks at a time, or the raw intensity of a full weekend of live events, I have to allow myself to regroup mentally. You need to be OK with that and grant yourself the space you deserve in order to get back to your plan fully primed for more progress.

I had so, so many Sanctionals in the diary in the coming months, all of which I had booked as an insurance policy just in case I didn't actually receive the national champion invite. Filthy 150 was taking place in Ireland at the end of November, so only four weeks after the end of the 2019 Open. It seemed like it was right around the corner and neither my body nor mind were anywhere near ready for that, so I pulled out of the competition.

After a couple of weeks, I started at least making it into the gym and doing some training, although not with any sort of plan. I would just work on what I felt like on that day, sometimes making things up as I went along, or I'd jump in with one of the classes for a while and then drift off for stretch or just chat to one of our members. I deliberately avoided pushing myself and concentrated on getting my body moving, elevating my heart rate and having a bit of fun. It helped to take my mind off the constant worry of whether I would really be going to the Games or not.

Otherwise, I would have been stressing about it all day, every day. I was watching and re-watching my Open workout videos to check if all my reps were OK, wondering if I'd properly locked out at the top of a movement or satisfied the standards that CrossFit published for each event and I would text Ben screen shots asking him if he thought a particular squat was low enough or if I'd stood up straight at the top of a box jump. He would always tell me they were all fine and I should try to chill out. I had to coach myself to forget what I had achieved and it was a weird feeling.

Two months after collapsing off the rower at the end of the fifth Open workout, I *finally* got confirmation that it was all official. I checked my phone in bed one morning and found I had an email saying all the scores had been verified or adjusted and I had been invited to the CrossFit Games as the national champion of the UK. I got up and went to the gym as normal.

I felt extremely proud that I'd achieved a goal that I had worked towards for so long. I was proud of the hard work I'd put in and of the seven years of progress – as a person as well as an athlete. And yet, although it felt good to get that validation, I couldn't help but be a bit disappointed that I missed out on an initial sense of celebration. But I realised that, in the grand scheme of things, it didn't take away from how it felt to be officially the fittest in the UK and it is something that I will cherish forever.

Still, though, that eight weeks of limbo was one of the strangest periods of my life. When you go to a live competition, you know at the end of the weekend exactly where you've finished. At the Regionals in Berlin the year before, when my main focus was to enjoy myself and dance around after each event, I didn't have to wait for that feeling of completion. Now, after the biggest achievement of my career to date, I was listless and really unmotivated.

I had always classed myself as extremely mentally strong and if I was determined to do something I'd just get on with it. So, after the Open I thought I would get straight back to training and go even harder. That I would be able to push through and start nailing my weaknesses. In actual fact, that two months showed me that you can have a totally bullet-proof mindset and be a supremely driven person but you still need to give yourself a break.

It's like trying to jump back up for a second set of pull-ups before you're ready, or like back when I was trying to go unbroken on the toes-to-bar in my first local CrossFit competition and had to stop because my abs were cramping like crazy. Sometimes you can grit your teeth and manage a few more. But they will hurt like hell and, trust me, you will redline soon after and not be able to do another rep, no matter how much you want to or how hard you try. I had mentally redlined.

I don't regret that experience because it will make me a better athlete, businessperson, friend and partner. If you know you're not totally on it and that you can't commit fully to something completely at that moment, it's right to take a break. More than that, you *must* take a break. As long as you know that you're doing so in order to start moving forward again with a renewed passion, you won't lose sight of your goal. Just as with pacing a workout, planned rest is always the smartest strategy.

GIVE YOURSELF A BREAK

When you're busy working on a project, in the office, at home or in the gym, it is all too easy to convince yourself that you simply don't have time to take any breaks at all. But even small breaks can be extremely beneficial to your performance.

A study published in the *Journal of Occupational Health Psychology* found that regular breaks have a positive impact on your wellbeing, increasing energy levels and decreasing exhaustion. Longer breaks, classed as 45 minutes or more, lunchtime breaks of 30 minutes and even micro-breaks of 10 minutes or less can all reduce stress, maintain your performance and limit the need for longer recovery at the end of the day.

The simplest way to adapt to taking micro-breaks is by being more conscious of your own level of focus. Next time you find yourself distracted from the project in hand – surfing the internet on your laptop while working or scrolling through social media when you're sorting something at home – set the timer on your phone for five minutes. When the alarm goes off, get back onto your task.

> You may well find these breaks happen every hour or so, or even every half an hour. Everyone is different but the key is to keep them short. Set that timer as soon as you realise your focus has wandered and you'll reap the rewards.

Once I felt like I had taken enough time to recuperate and re-energise, I had to go straight into a full-on block of competition training to prepare for the Dubai CrossFit Championship in December. The event in Dubai has been one of the marquee comps of the season for years and always attracts the biggest of the big-name athletes with the quality of workouts, how well they look after the competitors and, of course, a massive prize purse. I already had an invite to the Games in hand but it was the first opportunity for Sam and I to travel as part of the new CrossFit season; I would be able to test myself against some of the very top athletes and we'd have the opportunity to explore such a different culture.

The events in Dubai are renowned for being as intense and varied as those at the Games and it was a good chance for me to experience that ahead of going to Madison. There was swimming and sandbag work and brand new movements that I'd not performed before at a live event. We did sprint workouts that were over in less than 90 seconds and a chipper with a 15-minute time limit. I also had the opportunity to test myself against athletes like Patrick Vellener, Brent Fikowski and Bjorvin Karl Gudmundsson, all of whom have recently stood on the podium at the CrossFit Games.

After any competition, it always takes you a little while to get back to proper training again because your body is battered. I had just established that it was better for me to have three to four weeks off after any competition but almost the moment I got back from Dubai, I had to move into prepping for CrossFit Strength in Depth, which was taking place in January. It's my favourite UK event and I wanted to perform and have fun in front of the crowd, as ever. To be able to do that at the Excel in London and for so many of my closest friends, my family and the CrossFit BFG community to be there is always special.

I had the confidence of being the UK's national champion but I knew my fitness wasn't anywhere near where it needed to be in either Dubai or at Strength in Depth, because I hadn't been training properly at all. Ben had to constantly remind me that we weren't there to win, that we knew I wasn't in peak condition and that I should just go out on the floor and enjoy myself. To commit to the moment. As a natural competitor and a professional athlete, it's always tricky to manage that inner fire and not go as hard as you can, though.

I finished fourteenth in Dubai and twelfth at Strength in Depth, both of which I was pleased with considering I was not in competition shape. The best result was to be able to take part without the desperate need to win, as I had my ticket to the Games already. Guys like David Shorunke needed to peak for those comps in the hunt for that coveted invite. David was successful and got a spot by finishing second at Strength in Depth, with the winner and multiple CrossFit Games champion Mat Fraser already qualified. I was hugely relieved not to have that pressure as it let me focus on having fun again.

The following month, February, Sam and I travelled to Miami for Wodapalooza, another of the most popular Sanctionals. I was meant to be competing but I was physically in bits again after Strength in Depth and carrying a few little niggles, so I withdrew. But Sam was taking part in one of the divisions, so I went to support her, have a good time and soak in the sunshine and atmosphere. The plan was to knuckle down when I got back and start building for the CrossFit Games, taking place at the end of July. I felt ready to start dialling up my training and was excited about taking my fitness to the next level, but in Miami, I could relax and enjoy being in the crowd for once. It turned out to be an amazing holiday.

SET ASIDE SOME TIME

If you experience any hurdles – and when you're working towards a goal you almost certainly will – it is important that you give yourself some mental space to process your feelings. But setting a time limit on that stage of disappointment is vital and it can encourage you to start evaluating the setback more logically.

How long you will need is entirely personal and dependant on the sort of setback you've experienced. It might be as little as an hour or as much as months. The best rule of thumb is to set your time limit, then add a bit extra. Even if you feel ready to move on before the time is up, be strict with yourself and wait it out.

If you've been working towards eating a healthier diet but have slipped up and eaten junk food all weekend, it's fine to be a bit annoyed with yourself. By giving yourself a day to sit with that feeling and then turn the page, you will find yourself with renewed motivation. The extra energy and willpower you'll have to get cracking is always worth it.

When we got home from Miami mid-February, I had that buzz again, my body felt amazing and I started to properly push during my training sessions. I was already ramping up nicely and a few of us sat down and drew up a proper plan with a series of training blocks that would take me all the way up to the Games, factoring in more of the Games-specific disciplines that almost always play a big part in Madison, like longer-distance running, open-water swimming and working with odd objects, such as heavy sandbags or weighted sleds.

There were rumours regarding a virus that was doing the rounds in China and popping up in a few other countries in that part of the world. We chatted about it at the gym and I genuinely thought that if there was going to be a lockdown like everyone was saying, then it would be one of those things that was over in a few weeks and we'd be back to normal. Then, as the cases around the world and in the UK spiralled upwards, the country locking down entirely looked very likely. Even when we had to shut the gym, we thought we'd be open again in a couple of weeks. Maybe a month at most? How wrong we were.

Ben texted me to say that the Olympics were going to be cancelled and that he doubted the CrossFit Games would take place. I felt like by July, things might be all right, so I worked out as best as I could at home with kit that I'd picked up from the gym but I was as unsure about the new normal as anyone else. I considered myself extraordinarily lucky to live in a nice house with Sam and have everything we needed to keep safe, well fed and in training.

Over the months that followed, the CrossFit Games began to change shape. Because of the ban on large-scale sports events in the USA, it was announced that spectators would not be allowed and it was going to be just athletes and coaches on site. That made a massive difference to how I was mentally approaching that season. Such a huge part of getting to the Games, of achieving my goal, was to be able to celebrate and share it with my family and friends. It wasn't going to be the same without the people closest to me, the people who had sacrificed so much to get me there.

So I was already mentally preparing myself for change and I felt like whatever happened next wasn't a big deal, I was going to roll with it. I would compete anyway but I was determined to get to the Games again the year after, so I could compete at that level when everyone was there with me.

In April, it was announced that CrossFit HQ were looking at the option of holding the event at a ranch in Aromas, California, owned by the family of the director of the CrossFit Games, Dave Castro, and that they were also considering the possibility of some or all of the competition taking place in a virtual format. Then, in early May, the next alterations were released. I was having a romantic meal at home with Sam and we'd agreed not to have our phones at the dinner table but mine kept buzzing away in the other room, so I went to have a quick look. Loads and loads of people were tagging me into a post by the CrossFit Games Instagram account which detailed the latest changes to the event. That's how I found out that I was no longer going to live out my dream.

They had rescinded the invitations extended to the 239 national champions and were cutting the field down to the top 20 from the Open and the winners of the 10 Sanctionals that had taken place before the world went into lockdown. I had finished twenty-sixth on the global leader board. I had lost my golden ticket.

MAKE DISAPPOINTMENT YOUR ALLY

Research published in the journal *Nature* has found proof that setbacks do lead to greater success in the future. The study authors compared scientists who just missed out on a professional grant with those who just succeed, then observed their careers for a ten-year period.

Some of the 'near-miss' group did leave the industry almost immediately. But of the remaining 'near-miss' and 'near-win' scientists, those who did not get the first grant consistently outperformed their initially more successful colleagues. They had received just as much funding in the long term, published more papers and won more awards. The results showed that those who'd had that first setback overtook their peers who hadn't. It was that failure and the mental strength gained from the experience that led to their success over time.

Their conclusion was that failure is not simply an unavoidable reality of striving to achieve your goals but a valuable tool for future success. In fact, if you fail it increases your chances of being more successful in the long term.

159

Consider when in your life you've taken an easier route to avoid something that you believed would trip you up. Maybe you've been offered a new job but decided to play it safe and stay where you are as you knew the ropes, or even opted not to do some home improvements because you didn't think you would do a good enough job.

It makes sense to fail and your best bet for success is to fail often. Take the new job and if it doesn't work out, you know more about the roles that would really suit you. Give the DIY a go and should you make a mistake, you'll get the hang of it for next time.

As you are driving towards your goal, try to embrace the harder path sometimes, rather than taking the easier route. Each speed bump will only further smooth the road ahead.

Sam was absolutely fuming that I'd been cut from the Games. I've not seen her like that, ever. My family and friends were all gutted for me and my support team were furious but I was fine. I know that sounds weird but I was honestly OK with it and thought to myself, 'This is out of my control – what's the point in stressing out about it?' All the experiences that had forged the Start Where Others Stop mindset – my struggles with my weight as a kid and the abrupt end of my rugby ambitions; the meteoric rise of my personal training business and the dramatic fall of Be Fitter Gym; missing out on becoming national champion and then redeeming myself the next year – I always thought were all part of the journey to get me to the Games and cross that goal off my board. But they weren't.

It turned out that all of that had actually been preparing me for the moment I checked my phone and found out that I was no longer going to the 2020 Crossfit Games as the UK's national champion. Before I'd even taken a breath, I had already mentally flipped the switch and started focusing on the positives. I saw it as being given a six-month off season to put more energy into other areas of my life and explore new opportunities with work and sponsors. I would not have time to explore any of that if I was training and resting on repeat for the biggest competitive event of my life.

When I looked at it through that prism of my mindset, I was able to understand that I could not change what had happened. You only have the power to influence your own response to external events and the terrible impact of a pandemic on millions of people around the world was not something that I or anyone else could even start to contemplate having any control over.

I realised that I *had* achieved my dream and that was a truth that could not be taken away from me. I simply didn't get to experience the dream in full and that was OK because

I was going to get back there and ensure I was fitter, stronger, faster and more skilled than I'd ever been.

The next morning, I woke up and ate the same breakfast I always do. I threw on some kit and headed to the gym with Sam. We put on some music and warmed up, then we started training for the 2021 CrossFit Games.

YOUR SWOS PROGRAMME

Once you have set aside some time to allow the disappointment of a setback take its course, then started to comprehend how failure is a contributor to success that is actually worth embracing, you are ready for the last part of this section of your Start Where Others Stop Programme – how to make a comeback!

There are simple steps you can take to help you evaluate, process and plan to not just get up off the canvas but come back swinging. You should be used to this format by now, so use the exercise template on page 236 or grab your notebook and here we go:

CONSIDER ALL THE ANGLES

Even after you've gained some objectivity after the flashpoint of the failure, it is possible to fixate upon something you did or failed to do. But it may well be another factor that was not directly under your control.

If you failed to land your dream job even though you felt like you interviewed quite well, perhaps they hired internally to save on the salary. While it is valid to look at your own performance, other forces may have contributed. Make a note of all and everything you can think of that may have led to your setback – whether that's internal of external.

BE A 'SITUATION' SOLVER

The more you can move away from an emotional response, the better your comeback will be. Rather than basing your planning on making yourself feel better, start by thinking about what the situation requires. Immediately applying for another job feeds your emotional need to put disappointment behind you but maybe the situation dictates that you need more experience or a new qualification. This time, write down what practical steps you can take to improve. As we covered earlier, micro-goals are the aim here. Think back to what you learned in Chapter Two, when we practised breaking larger goals into smaller chunks. Now we're going to apply that same thinking to bouncing back from failure.

FOCUS ON TOMORROW

Take into account all that you've evaluated from your setback. Finally, look over your list of steps and make a note of what single thing you can do tomorrow to start making progress. If you let yourself become overawed by the long-term notion of making a comeback you may find yourself faced with the same risk of procrastination we overcame at the beginning of this book. Begin with tomorrow and get started.

PART III

ACHIEVE ANYTHING

CHAPTER SEVEN

FIND YOUR COMMUNITY

Since I started competing in CrossFit, I have done so as an individual. Compared to rugby, which is one of the most team-oriented of sports, when I enter a competition it is only my name on the starting mat beneath my feet, it is Zack George you can find in the final standings. My sponsors have come on board because they believe in me – my ability and my personality.

It's not just me though, of course. I have Sam, without whom I wouldn't get through a single day, and I have my trusted crew at the gym, who train with me and keep me motivated when I'm not totally feeling it. I have Harmeet and Josh, who handle all the coaching and are always there when I'm formulating a new strategy for a workout or trying to plan a better way to improve upon my fitness. I have Ben, who crunches the numbers and looks after the logistics at competitions so I can just go out and perform. It really does take a village.

I have also always been able to rely upon the unwavering support of my wider CrossFit BFG family, whose cheers and screams during Open events have given me the extra push I need to truly pour everything I have into the most horrible of workouts. I consider some of my fellow competitors good friends and at live competitions I look forward to catching up with them in the warm-up area. Even though we all want to beat one another when the buzzer sounds, before and after it's all smiles.

Finally, there is CrossFit in and of itself. People start coming to get in shape, lose weight or build a bit of muscle, sure, but they almost always stay for the community. From the very top of the sport to the 6 a.m. class on a Tuesday at your local box, we all celebrate one another's victories, be that a first pull-up, a 100kg snatch or being crowned the UK national champion. You may be in your fifties doing your first session, or a teenager just looking for a group of people to connect with – we're all in it together. We all stay and cheer until the last person finishes a workout.

During a three-week period in June 2020, all of those communities were tested by painful controversy, one that would change the shape of CrossFit once again. It was proof that if you want to be successful, you need the support of people you value and trust. It doesn't matter if your goal is to get in shape, spend more time with your children or cut down on your drinking. Our goals are ours and ours alone. But together, we can achieve anything.

When George Floyd died while being arrested in Minneapolis on 25 May 2020, there was an overwhelming surge of protests calling for an end to racial inequality around the world. On Saturday 6 June 2020, CrossFit's founder and CEO Greg Glassman posted a racially insensitive remark on Twitter replying to a University of Washington Institute tweet that described racism and discrimination as public health issues. Glassman's response was 'It's: FLOYD-19'.

The CrossFit community immediately condemned the remarks. Hundreds of gyms around the world ended their official affiliation and brands associated with the company, of which Glassman was the 100 per cent owner. Brands such as Reebok, who had been the title sponsor of the CrossFit Games for a decade, immediately distanced themselves from Glassman and CrossFit.

Again, I found out about it all when people started tagging me into posts on Instagram and my friends began messaging me to ask if I'd seen what Glassman had said. To start with, I thought it was a joke, or a meme, or that one of my mates was playing a practical joke on me. It was so wrong I was *sure* somebody was winding me up. Once I started looking into it though, I realised it was true – that was what he had actually said. Immediately I felt angry and annoyed but then a fraction of a second later, I also felt disappointed and let down. My dream had been to compete at the Games and I had made it my life to get there. For him to crush seven years

171

of hard, painful work in one tweet was gutting. I felt like he had destroyed the sport of CrossFit in 140 characters or less.

It took me a couple of hours to compute the whole thing. It was difficult to comprehend. For someone like Glassman, who was in such a powerful position as the leader of a global business, to come out with such an insensitive and inflammatory remark simply didn't make sense to me. When I had come to terms with the fact that he had actually made those comments, I messaged my agent James and told him I couldn't be a part of CrossFit if the CEO owner had those views. At that moment, I felt like my time with CrossFit was over and, in the immediate aftermath of Glassman's comments, I felt as though CrossFit was going to die. It didn't seem to me like there was any chance of it coming back from the firestorm that was quickly developing unless he sold the company and cleared off and, frankly, I couldn't see him doing that. I remember thinking that there was no way Glassman was going to give up his ownership of CrossFit. He struck me as so power mad that I couldn't see anything changing. I thought to myself, 'We're going to have to find a new sport to get our teeth into.' It was like the rug had been pulled out from beneath our feet and it was deeply upsetting.

What especially hurt was not just that his comments were wildly offensive on a human level but also that I had poured so much time and effort into a sport where the CEO felt comfortable enough to make those remarks – it was unbelievably demoralising. I am one of the few Black athletes at the top level of the sport and the nature of the tweet was hugely hurtful. I think the vast majority of Black people would have felt very offended by it. So for me, it was not just my dreams and time spent dedicated to the sport that had been shattered but, as a Black man, I was angry. I was really worried that people would let this just blow over and he could get away with it, only for something to happen again six months down the line.

I've never felt intimidated or unwelcome because of the colour of my skin at CrossFit, so in a way his comments were even more irritating. I've never been involved in or even anywhere near any sort of confrontation because of my or somebody else's race. I've trained in CrossFit gyms around the world and I've not given a second thought to walking into any of them. I feel confident that I never will. But when Glassman showed such ignorance of a worldwide situation and put out an insensitive message without understanding the incredible pain it would cause, I thought it sent a terribly bad message. Anyone seeing that tweet from outside of the CrossFit sphere could assume that his views were representative of what most of the people who do CrossFit think. That the majority of us probably have those same views. The possibility of this really hurt.

There is no denying that the sport is predominantly white. Membership at a CrossFit box tends to be fairly expensive, so there are socio-economic factors to bear in mind, as the cost of joining a gym can be prohibitive to less privileged people. While reaching less privileged groups is something that could be addressed by the company moving forwards, I have never personally felt uncomfortable in any sort of situation in the sport on account of my skin colour.

I had never seen myself as a role model and I still don't, even though I know I sort of am in a sense. I have never consciously thought about how much of an impact I might make but I was in such a unique position after Glassman's comments, as an elite Black athlete and box owner. I felt like I really wanted to own that and live up to it, so, at that time, more than ever, I realised I had an opportunity to be a vocal figure that people could look up to. To be a voice demanding change.

I wanted it to be known that – as a Black guy in CrossFit and someone who competes at a high level – I had not come across any sort of racial abuse. Glassman's tweet doesn't reflect the community's views and outlook, which are inclusive and progressive in many ways. I wanted anyone who's not into CrossFit to know that this simply isn't how our community operates and I wanted them to know that the CrossFit community is a place for *everyone*, no matter the colour of their skin.

In the workouts programmed in every gym, at levels of competition, from local throwdowns to the CrossFit Games, while the weight, calories and reps are adjusted for men and women to reflect the undeniable biological differences between male and female bodies, we all complete the same movements. We all do the same workout. The prizes on offer for those taking part have always been the same regardless of gender (unlike other sports, such as tennis or football, for example) and athletes become fan favourites purely on the basis of their characters, rather than gender, race or sexuality. Many events – like Wodapalooza in Miami, most notably – host competitions for less able athletes, with the movements adapted for each person to create a level playing field regardless of their individual requirements. Watching a person in a wheelchair doing pull-ups or an army veteran who has lost an arm lifting a barbell with one hand is massively inspiring.

Elite athletes began to announce that they would be boycotting the CrossFit Games in condemnation of Glassman's comments, including former champions and those who have stood on the podium. I immediately made it very clear on social media and in interviews over the next few days that even if I were to end up being invited to the Games, I would decline my spot. Although our stance might have seemed extreme, it was the only course of action for me. Even though I had grafted for seven years, I would not sacrifice my morals. I would not be competing again in an event run by CrossFit Inc. unless Greg Glassman stepped down. I felt so strongly about withdrawing my support from a company who had a leader with those views. Hundreds of CrossFit gyms around the world, who all pay CrossFit an annual fee to use the brand name and training methodology, began to cancel their affiliation. Many changed their names to remove any reference to CrossFit at all.

I think it was the first time that we, as athletes, stood together and made our power known. We simply weren't going to let him say whatever he wanted and get away with it. There had been rumblings of discontent the year before, when Glassman initiated the wholesale changes to the competitive season without any empathy for the professional competitors it directly impacted. Allegations of Glassman being guilty of repeated sexist behaviour and remarks soon surfaced. So too did an email exchange with the female owner of a gym that had been affiliated for nine years, who wrote to Glassman to explain why his tweet and the lack of adequate remorse meant she was going to de-affiliate. He accused her of having mental health issues.

Even the easy-to-overlook fact that many of the benchmark workouts had been given female names by Glassman, like the Linda workout I performed back at the European regional in Berlin, now took on a slightly uncomfortable edge. When asked why he did so, he is widely quoted as having said, 'Anything that leaves you flat on your back, looking up at the sky asking, "What just happened to me?" deserves a female's name.'

An apology was put out by the company on behalf of Glassman but it was very slow in being published and rang hollow when it was. The feeling was that it was nowhere near good enough and there was renewed demand for real change. On 9 June, it was announced that Greg Glassman was stepping down but, while it was a move in the right direction, he was still the 100 per cent owner and, as result, would benefit from gym affiliation fees or people paying to register for the Open. I for one was still not going to support CrossFit if he was still going to be raking in profit. He needed to be cut out of the organisation completely by selling all of his shares.

Again, the community was unified in our response. Big-name athletes felt the same way I did: like this was a sham of an exit and he needed to be completely removed, not just from the running of the CrossFit but as the beneficiary of the financial success of the company, too.

I was contacted by many of the top competitors who contend for the CrossFit Games on a regular basis and received notes from other athletes saying that they were so happy that I had made a stand. I think people really appreciated that I was not fearful of saying what I felt. Some people in our position and with our platform are worried about annoying certain people or losing followers on social media, which paralyses them and stops them making any sort of change.

I was not concerned about that. I wasn't worried about anyone saying my views were too strong or that I shouldn't be voicing them. I felt like it was my duty to speak up. I had one of the biggest platforms in UK CrossFit, both in terms of followers on social media and being the UK's number one athlete; I had name recognition at the highest level of the sport; I was one of the few elite Black athletes *and* I was the owner of a CrossFit gym, so I was in the unique position of being affected on every level. I felt proud to voice my opinion.

I wanted to be somebody who people could look up to and feel like their national champion was making a stand.

I had direct messages from individuals and gyms thanking me for representing the UK CrossFit scene. Most people don't have the platform to make their views heard. By speaking out, I tried to provide the British CrossFit community with a voice that would be impossible to ignore.

BE A QUIET LEADER

Very few goals we set ourselves are truly individual. Whether you're training for success in sport, like I am, or striving for a better salary in your professional life, how you interact with the other people who are directly or indirectly tied into your progress can give you a real advantage. When you are in a position of even slight authority, those people will look to you for leadership.

But you don't have to be an extrovert to become a leader. In fact, being somebody who can encourage others to speak up can be inspiring in a more inclusive way. To be a 'quiet leader', you just need to create an environment where your friends, colleagues, teammates or clients feel confident and empowered to voice their opinions and put forward their ideas.

How you do this is simple: you listen. Quiet leaders tend to listen more than they talk and when they do speak, it is when they have something important to add. Next time you want to interrupt while someone else is speaking, try subtly standing or sitting in a way that allows you to place a finger over your lips. It sounds extreme but that physical cue will stop you thinking about what you want to say and allow you to zone back in on what is being said instead.

Quiet leaders are also generally more reflective, taking time to reach an opinion rather than making snap judgements. Listen to people, take your time, then talk when you've got something worth saying. That is the best way to lead by example.

There was a choice to be made about the future of Cross-Fit BFG. With so many gyms de-affiliating and dropping the 'CrossFit' part of their brand names as a result of Glassman's comments, it would have been easy for me to follow suit and break ties between the businesses. But we think of ourselves as a family and there was no doubting that it had to be a group decision.

I messaged our members group on Facebook and laid out our options, as although everyone knew where I stood on a personal level and had been hugely supportive, I wanted this to be a choice we made together. My thoughts were that we should hold fire on making a snap decision about de-affiliation and to see how things played out over the next few weeks. I explained that, in my opinion, we could do with being patient, because if CrossFit made the changes demanded by the wider community, we would wish we hadn't ended our affiliation.

I was so proud of the CrossFit BFG family. I had taken a strong position as an individual but the team and all the members decided upon a sensible approach. Many people and a lot of gyms were making this huge call on the direction of their businesses and their own communities from a place of anger, which I found completely understandable as I was angry, too. But it wasn't just about me, it was about our Leicester-based community and they all valued the chance to voice their thoughts on the issues we were all trying to come to terms with.

We chose, as a gym, to wait. We were going to bide our time and see what happened rather than rush into a decision. We agreed that nobody condoned Glassman's comments or behaviour but that did not reflect who we were as a group. We voted unanimously to remain affiliated until the dust had settled, conscious that we all needed more time to process what had happened. Everyone was willing to give CrossFit a chance to make the right changes.

On 24 June 2020, it was announced that Glassman was selling 100 per cent of the company. It was a powerful example that we as athletes can determine what happens to the sport to which we devote our lives. For us to demand change and for that to have an effect was a positive beacon in what was otherwise an extremely dark time for the sport. I was proud of the impact that we, as a community, were able to have and how we trusted one another to react in the right way. We had faith in the leaders of our communities to make their stand, to ensure those without a real voice were heard loud and clear. I believed that those in my communities, from the elite athletes and the multinational brands, to our UK scene and especially our tight-knit CrossFit BFG tribe, would all say what needed saying and do what needed to be done.

Placing your trust in people who share your goals or values can be a massively positive force for change of any kind. In almost every area of your life, trusting those who align with your hunger for improvement makes a huge difference to your likelihood of success. On a simple level, it's why having a training partner who also wants to transform their fitness makes it much more likely that you will both succeed. You have to trust one another to turn up to every session and the positive feedback loop that creates is extremely powerful: neither of you miss workouts, therefore you make progress faster, which means you want to keep turning up. And on and on it goes.

WIDEN YOUR CIRCLE

Closely monitoring your progress towards a goal is a proven method of increasing your likelihood of success. But new research by the University of Sheffield states that you have to monitor the behaviour you wish to change and it is crucial in long-term success.

The study's authors undertook a meta-analysis of nearly 20,000 participants to look at the effectiveness of prompts to monitor their progress towards a number of goals, mainly concentrating on losing weight, changing diet and stopping smoking. Their results showed that you must be specific – those who wanted to lose weight saw decreased success if they monitored their diet but an increase if they weighed themselves.

They also found that a vital component of success was not only monitoring your results but recording them and reporting them publicly. This can be as simple as starting a group chat with friends or colleagues who share your goal. If a few of you at work are training for a half-marathon, record your runs and report them to the group to see an increase in everyone's motivation and ultimate achievement.

We all have communities around us at work and at home and, in addition, our attitudes and interests connect us with even more. Being a fan of a football team, for example, links you not only to the many others who support that team but also the hundreds of millions of football fans around the world. You may not feel those connections on a daily basis, or even be aware of them. But if one day your team's owner fired the very popular manager or the governing body changed the rules of football entirely, you would feel those bonds instantly and realise that they had been there all along.

Two weeks after Glassman resigned, the company was officially bought outright by Eric Roza, a former CrossFit affiliate owner and the founder of a data and analytics company. Roza came with a track record of fostering inclusive and understanding working environments, which, combined with his personal experience of running a CrossFit box, made him a solid fit to start fixing the wounds of not only the last few weeks but the past few years under the previous regime.

It was a good change and the final step I needed to say that I was back behind CrossFit and I could completely believe in the brand and the sport. More than that, I felt like I was ready to compete and keep progressing as an athlete because, as I saw it, the right decisions were made. Granted, they could have been made faster and the communication with the community during those tense weeks probably could have been more open and transparent but these are all areas for growth for the company under Roza's guidance. Only time will tell if he's able to take CrossFit in the right direction.

One thing that might help is the formation of a governing body that upholds the rules and regulations of competition as well as handling all athlete matters, such as the quality of judging, the process of appealing decisions during events and testing for performance enhancing drugs. As athletes, we approach training, competing and all the countless hours, days, weeks and months of hard work as professionals – we need to evolve into an official sport, like rugby or football.

On a wider level, I feel like addressing how expensive CrossFit can be is a clear route to progress. It will always, and should always, be priced higher than a commercial gym, because you're getting coached by experts who are programming specifically for you and your local community, rather than just paying to use the equipment. But there are ways of making it more accessible to the less privileged and engaging a wider spectrum of society. CrossFit could go into lower income areas around the world and offer seminars and workshops for free. The price of affiliating a gym has always been fixed but being able to scale that to an appropriate level according to the financial conditions of a particular area would make opening a box in less affluent areas more viable. Perhaps the coaching courses could be offered at a much lower price to encourage the creation of local communities that might not even exist in a gym but who meet somewhere with a few bits of kit to train hard every day and have a good time while getting healthier and fitter.

I've always said the best thing about CrossFit is the sense of community. At any box, it doesn't matter what age, gender or sex you are or how fit or unfit you are; regardless of what colour, shape or size you come in, you will be welcomed. There will be alternatives for every movement for the day's session on the whiteboard and you will be able to get just as good a workout as the elite athlete training next to you. It becomes a place where you socialise, where you meet new friends or even partners and you look forward to going to the box every single day of every single week.

It is so different to going into a normal gym, sticking some headphones in so you don't have to speak to anyone, going through the motions and not really know what you're doing. The community in CrossFit is always there and it travels all the way from your local box up to the highest level of the sport. Even on the competition floor, you see the athletes supporting one another as they push themselves to the very limit of human capacity.

In the last throes of Glassman's reign, the internal media teams were drastically cut as he wanted to downplay the emphasis on the top athletes and the Games as a whole. But it is the documentaries and videos they produced that got so, so many people into the sport. It was that video on YouTube of the athletes looking ripped before the workout in the pool that got me into CrossFit in the first place, after all. So I feel like bringing that back is something that would both serve and grow the community.

People who play five-a-side football once a week all love watching the Premiership. They know they aren't going to play for Manchester City but many are still obsessed with the sport and are motivated by the abilities of the top players in the world. That's what keeps them playing. Tennis courts around the UK are all booked out for weeks after Wimbledon has been on TV for the same reason – we are inspired by the best in the world to become a bit better ourselves.

I know that I am willing to give Roza and his team the time they need to make progress. If they can overcome their hurdles and turn their weakness into strengths; if they can win back the trust of the community, then they'll be on the right track. My path is to the 2021 CrossFit Games, so I guess I'll see them on the road.

The falling of the house of cards and the dawn of the new ownership capped off a complicated couple of months after what had felt like a long and extremely turbulent year. Throughout it all, Sam has always been there for me, doing whatever she thinks she needs to do to support me. Her reaction to the national champions being cut from the Games that evening, when we were having our date night, was incredible. I'm such a laid-back guy and generally pretty chilled but her fury and outrage was her way of showing me how much my dream had become our dream

When it was officially announced that the top 20 from the Open and the ten Sanctional qualifiers were going to compete in an online competition, with only the top five men and women going to California to compete in person, and that, barring a bizarre slew of injuries, I would categorically *not* be going to the Games, I was honestly relieved. Even after all the alterations to the structure and schedule of the event, there was still a glimmer of hope that I might be able to compete in some form or another. Knowing where I stood was empowering and I could fully enjoy an off season and treat myself to some sweets and chocolate when I fancied it before I started gearing up for the coming season in October or November.

My family were upset that they weren't going to be able to watch me compete. But they knew that I'm willing to put in the work to get there even more convincingly next time, so they were behind me, as ever. I've always had such great support from my close family and friends, who have been there for me through all my ups and downs. That has never, and will never, be in doubt.

The new backing I have felt from the whole CrossFit community is something I will always be massively grateful for. People I've never met are urging me forwards, telling me I deserve to be at the Games because they've seen my journey over the years. I've tried to be honest about my progress and post both good and bad workouts on social media, and I receive messages of encouragement from my followers every day – so much so that it feels like they've been on the journey with me.

No matter how committed you are to achieving your dream, you need to surround yourself with good people – those who will tell you when you should knuckle down as well as when you could do with giving yourself a break, who will give you their hand if you stumble or even remove a hurdle or two from your path altogether if they can. The Start Where Others Stop mentality does not mean becoming a lone wolf, hungrily running on and on. It means finding a pack who are all going the same way and working together to chase down your collective goals. If one of you falls behind, you don't relentlessly plough ahead. You go back and get them. You pick them up.

CrossFit is a gruesome sport to do on your own. During lockdown in the UK, when it was announced that elite athletes in any sport could go and train in their own facilities, Sam would come to the gym with me every day. It was just me and her. Having someone there kept me motivated and without Sam I would have found training incredibly tough. When we do have our whole crew together, the power of our community is palpable – I have Ben and Dan Wagner, my main training partner, constantly thinking of new ways to perform a workout or a more efficient way to perform a movement. It is almost *always* a much better idea than I would have come up with on my own.

In competition, the support I have from Sam and my family is what makes the real difference. If I have a bad event, I just want to sulk, but my pack helps me up. They tell me that it's just one workout and that I have to put it behind me and focus on performing to my best ability in the next one. That each rep is a chance to prove I'm ready for the CrossFit Games. They remind me that I'm one of the best in the world. They pick me up. They make me believe in myself.

YOUR SWOS PROGRAMME

Having a community that supports you is amazing and a massive advantage when striving for a specific goal. But it is a two-way street – to truly unlock the mutually rewarding benefits of community, you have to be able to support other people when they need it. A full guide on how to offer support would require another book by another person but there are a few pitfalls that you can avoid in order to more empathetically provide somebody with a sense of community. Check out page 238 for some prompts to help you think about the below more thoroughly.

DON'T MAKE THEM ASK FOR HELP

Many people, even though they desperately want assistance with a particular issue or problem, are reluctant to ask for it. After all, voicing that an aspect of your life is not under control is hard. Offering your help is good;

offering detailed ways in which you can help is even better. If a family member is struggling with childcare arrangements, rather than just saying you'll help, suggest the days and times you can take care of the kids and some activities you could do with them.

DON'T MAKE IT ABOUT YOU

It's tempting to listen to what somebody is trying to tell you about their personal situation and then reply by relating it to your own experiences. This is a slight misunderstanding of empathy, however. Saying 'I know exactly how you feel' is always done with good intentions but it can serve to minimise their emotions or issues. Instead, listen and let them be honest about how they feel. And then listen some more for good measure.

DON'T FORGET THE PERSON

Any advice you might come across when it comes to giving support to somebody else, including the above, should never be considered an accurate or exhaustive guide. Every person is different and the community they may require will differ according to the person and the context. Just because a certain method of support was valued by somebody previously, it doesn't mean that it's right for another person, or even for the same person in a different situation. Offer specific help, listen to what they need to say and then go from there.

Being a proactive source of care and support for the people around you is a genuinely rewarding practice that creates a positive feedback loop – your support engenders others to support you in a constantly refreshing cycle. Knowing that your community, no matter how big or small, is there for one another gives each member the belief that they can be themselves. The next chapter explores the power of that self-belief and how you can unlock the final pieces of the Start Where Others Stop mindset.

CHAPTER EIGHT

BUILD YOUR SELF-BELIEF

By this point, perhaps you've made some progress towards changing or improving yourself and broken it down into the steps you need to take to make it manageable. Hopefully you've enjoyed a few milestones and, if you've had a setback or two, you've found a way to reach even higher and put your trust in those who share your goal. There is one small but crucial element of the Start Where Others Stop mentality that remains, and you may well have come to realise this in your own journey: you have to find some self-belief.

It's an easy thing to say but it is much harder to truly put into practice. As humans, we are hard-wired to focus on the negatives and it's an evolutionary tool that has made us the dominant species on the planet. Our prehistoric ancestors concentrated on the things that could kill them, like 'do not eat the red berries', rather than 'those purple ones are really nice'. Obviously we don't find ourselves in that situation today but there are moments in your daily life that can be transformed by a bit of self-belief.

Take your work life, for example. Let's say you and your team are putting together an important project and you had an out-there idea with the potential to revolutionise the way you all work. It could bring in more profit or lead to more efficient use of time and resources. It's a good idea. But you are thrown off by doubt in yourself before you say anything. After all, you've never spoken up or voiced your opinions of how your company should operate, let alone emailed your boss about them. You just work there.

Believing in yourself will help you speak up. It can turn what would otherwise be a missed opportunity into a huge leap forward in your career and show that you're more than just an average employee, happy to do only what is asked of you and nothing more.

The same thinking applies when you're at home. Maybe you're having a few issues with your partner and you second-guess how to react or what to say and keep silent because it feels safer not to be vulnerable. But it only makes things worse and makes it far more likely that flashpoint will come up again and again. In the gym, just believing you can lift a certain weight is often the difference between hitting a new Personal Record (PR) or staying stuck where you are.

By getting started and setting a target towards something you are passionate about, committing to each stage of the process and using setbacks positively, then building a team of like-minded people who support you as much as you back yourself, you have done everything in your power to make your dream real. Now all you have to do is find that belief.

For me, that confidence in myself and my ability flows directly from my parents and what they have achieved in their lives. Being around that all the time when I was growing as a person had a hugely positive impact on my mindset and it continues to do so. They had a lot of things to deal with when they were young and the racial abuse they experienced, even when they were first dating, meant their relationship was far from straightforward, yet they persevered when so many others would have not.

For Dad, starting out in business was all a matter of self-belief and mental resilience. A Black man in that sort of industry was very rare in those days but he had faith he could become a success, rather than listening to the whispering voice inside or the shouting voices of others saying that he should settle for being a mechanic. That he wasn't going to make it. It all came down to the colour of his skin – people weren't used to seeing Black men being successful, so for him to cope with that attitude and pursue that path anyway took an enormous amount of willpower and belief. Mum also had her own hurdles to negotiate. Being with a Black man was not the norm back then and to start a company together will have turned heads for all the wrong reasons. That their business did so well early on was a direct result of the belief they had in one another and their shared goals.

Living in our first home, the same one they bought when they were 21, was proof in bricks and mortar of that self-assurance. That my parents had come from nothing and bought this massive house was an example of what can happen when you trust yourself to be successful, whatever it is that you choose to do.

It was the mantra that Dad made part of our upbringing. I remember so many times him telling me that we had to believe in ourselves, that anything you truly, truly want to achieve or conquer in your life is possible if you work at it. That you had to know, deep down, that you can achieve it if you have the right mindset. He constantly reassured me that, if I believed, I *could* be the best. My parents have never told me not to try something because it was a bit out of my reach, instead their mentality has always been to aim as high as you can and then work as hard as possible to get there.

Clearly, though, self-belief alone is not always enough to achieve your goals. Having the confidence to aim as high as you can means that if you don't quite get there, you will still have made huge strides and learned so much more from any stumbling blocks than if you had set your target lower.

My whole story is shot through with the proof of the power of self-belief, though at the time I often didn't realise I was using such a powerful tool for positive development. My childhood dream of becoming a professional rugby player, for example:

I knew I wanted to excel at something, for myself but also for my dad, because he was a very good sportsman. He could see I was talented and playing well when he was watching was a good feeling. There were obvious steps to take, from playing for my school teams to representing Leicestershire and then training with the Tigers Academy. When I started having the odd niggle, I was determined to keep on grinding, sure that I would get through it and keep rising through the ranks until I went pro.

The constant injuries to my ankles and knees, however, meant I didn't achieve that goal. But because I had aimed so high, I learned some extremely valuable lessons in the process. I discovered that my mindset was an incredibly formative force and that I could handle most setbacks with self-belief and a positive attitude. More importantly, I worked out that I hadn't really been playing for the love of rugby, I was doing it because I was good at it. That conclusion was pivotal for my development as a person. I had to find my way forward into a sporting career that excited me.

Personal training was an obvious direction to take. When I began working at Nuffield Health aged 18, getting people in shape and connecting with clients using my own experience of transforming my fitness was hugely satisfying. I set myself a new goal: to open my own chain of gyms. Again, I was aiming very high.

I established the steps I needed to take towards that dream and began working my way through them, starting with training a few people out of a tiny studio at my parents' house, then running fitness classes with a car full of kettlebells and only one person turning up, to packing out sports halls five nights a week. When we opened Be Fitter Gym it was a big milestone on my way to my end goal.

It is easy to get wrapped up and lost in your end goal, to be constantly focused on the finish line. It is important to dream big but it's equally vital to celebrate each milestone along the way as if you don't, what's the point? People say 'you've got to enjoy the process' but you can't do that if you won't allow yourself to stop and savour it. Whether you're working towards self-fulfilment or self-betterment, you have to take a moment to be grateful for the work that you put in; without those celebrations you will lose sight of the end. It is only by looking back at what we've achieved that we can adapt our plans and continue progressing. By stopping to breathe in what you have done in the last weeks, months or even years, you can also assess if you're still working towards the right goal. You will be able to establish whether the work you're putting in is making the right impact. It stands to reason that if you always have your head down, you can't check if you're still going the right way.

When I opened that first gym, my goal was to make Be Fitter a huge success and then open another and keep going until I had my own fitness empire, so I put my head down and went for it. Three years later, I looked up and realised I had been working 12-hour shifts for six days a week and was not enjoying it. As a result, the business was not working out.

That the commercial gym was not a storming success was, at the time, the worst thing I could possibly imagine. But with the help of my dad, I quickly saw that I had not failed, I had simply developed as a person between leaving school at 18 and shutting the doors of Be Fitter when I was 24. Six years is a long time and my focus had naturally shifted.

Opening CrossFit BFG down the road from that first gym only a few weeks later seemed like a fast process. Too fast, even. But it summed up my mentality of not being afraid to give things a go, of aiming high so that any failure is a form of success. I had learned so much from running and closing Be Fitter and I poured all of it into the next venture. My mistakes were just opportunities to do better next time. You could say that, in regard to my original goal of owning a gym chain, I had failed. But I wouldn't be on the path I am today had I not been through that experience.

It is only by believing in yourself that you can understand that failure can be a positive step towards achieving your goals. That faith in your ability to adapt and thrive can fully unlock the Start Where Others Stop mindset. Each misstep simply becomes a chance to take that breath, steady yourself and move forward with renewed energy, more sure than ever of your footing.

When I saw that first clip of the CrossFit Games on You-Tube and wrote the goal of getting to that level on my board, I could have set my sights lower and aimed to compete at local competitions. At the time, I was *nowhere* near Games standard, so it would have been safer to hedge my bets and aim for something more obviously achievable. A lot of people would have and that's completely understandable.

But for me, I had the self-belief to aim as high as possible, to the very top of the sport, in fact. Because even if I didn't reach that point, there would have been experiences, opportunities and other goals along the way. If you aim low, or you don't think you can achieve anything beyond a certain point, you will always be limiting yourself. You will miss out on all the opportunities that thinking a bit bigger would present. You won't realise that having a huge dream grants you the opportunity to celebrate every smaller achievement contained within. You won't understand that backing yourself is your best chance for success.

EXERCISE SOME BELIEF

The theory that physical fitness and mental health are intrinsically linked is a popular one but scientists are now starting to investigate the exact force at play. A study of over 600 students conducted by Joseph, Royce, Benitez and Pezkemi that was published in the journal *Quality of Life Research*, established a direct link between physical training activity and self-belief, with physical self-esteem found to be 'the most powerful mediating variable on quality of life'.

The key aspect for self-esteem is adherence. Sticking to a programme of physical activity has an exponentially positive effect on your perceived level of self-belief. This could be moderate, such as walking rather than taking the bus three days a week, or more vigorous, like going to the gym every morning. It is sticking to it that makes the most difference.

Whatever your personal goal is, especially if it isn't fitness-based, planning some regular time for any kind of movement, be that walking, stretching, yoga, gardening or working out, is a self-fulfilling action that will only benefit your well-being.

Finding the opportunity for growth in a moment in which you have fallen short of your own expectations is not an easy process. Let's be honest, it can be a painful one and when I missed out on winning the 2019 CrossFit Open, my Start Where Others Stop mindset had its sternest examination. To be so, so close to achieving my goal and having it slip through my fingers because of a single movement was heart-breaking. I sulked in the aftermath of each attempt at those handstand push-ups and submitting a score that I knew would cost me my ticket to the Games was torturous.

I could have dwelled on it and let it ruin the rest of the season and the one after but I very quickly saw it as a setback that could launch me higher than I'd ever been. I had worked on so many areas of my fitness and was very good in those disciplines and movements. While one exercise stopped me from achieving my goal, it was *only one* exercise. I knew I would crush handstand push-ups, practise them relentlessly, turn that weakness into a strength and be ready for next year.

In the meantime, I was determined to do as well as possible in the remaining workouts. I wanted to win them, to prove to everyone else that it was only that small weakness at strict handstand push-ups that had held me back. I could have given up on the other workouts or told myself I had reached the ceiling of my potential and that I should set the bar lower. But I believed I was good enough to make it to the Games and took this as an opportunity to make myself even better before I got there.

We all have areas in which we aren't as strong as others and I will never be amazing at strict handstand push-ups. But now I'm good for my size and I've brought the movement up to a level where it doesn't hinder my performance in a workout or limit my other abilities and I'm OK with that. You don't have to be the best at everything and we have to understand that weaknesses are part of being human. Everyone has things that come naturally to them and others that they struggle with. In sports that is obvious but it is just as relevant to the rest of your life. At work there will be tasks at which you complete with ease and some that are much trickier and you have to really apply yourself to master. Maybe you can take some parts of parenting in your stride but feel totally out of your depth in other ways. Perhaps you're really good with people you know but find it hard to talk to strangers. You've just got to be willing to work on these areas and not get too wrapped up in making *everything* perfect. You have to believe in yourself as a person with strengths unlike anyone else's.

Nowhere is that self-belief more powerful for me than in the gym. Olympic weightlifting is a huge part of CrossFit and we all like to max out and go for new personal records once in a while, and although you can have the muscular strength and good technique, the impact of believing you can lift the bar cannot be underestimated. It is vital. So many people walk up to the bar, psyche themselves out and walk away again, worried about all the things that could go wrong, or the risk of injuring themselves. Even when they reapproach the bar and attempt the lift, you know they aren't going to manage it. They know they aren't going to manage it.

If you stride up to that bar with confidence, with a mindset of self-belief, the entire lift will look different. You'll grip the bar tighter and brace your core harder. Your mind won't trip over the details and obsess over the various points of technique that could go wrong and you just lift it, even though the weight might be heavy for you. If you attack it with confidence, your chances of success are hugely multiplied.

When I'm working out with my training partners or coaching somebody, I will often not tell them how much weight I'm putting on the bar. Let's say they want to snatch 100kg and can lift 97.5kg but whenever they put on the extra 2.5kg they simply can't seem to do it. That three-digit number is playing tricks on them mentally and they talk themselves out of it before even taking hold of the bar.

If you don't tell them exactly what's on the bar and urge them to just get on and lift it, nine times out of ten they will execute it perfectly and they will be amazed that it was 100kg. If you let doubt creep in, it will always limit your potential, even in areas that you deem to be strengths. Believing that you are capable of more is one of the simplest tools to boost your performance in any sphere of your day-to-day life and one you can start using right now.

I believe I'm going to be the best male athlete in the UK in the 2021 CrossFit Open. I'm going to have my most dominant performance, set myself apart at the top of the UK leader board and I want to finish in the top ten globally. If the format of the season ever changes again, I will adapt and thrive in the stages required to qualify for the 2021 CrossFit Games and, when I get there, I am going to finish as the highest-ranking male UK athlete ever. Those are my goals and not a day passes when I don't think about them. Each workout is a step in the right direction, physically and mentally; every meal I eat and hour I sleep is a chance to get better. They are all a chance to believe.

I believe in myself. I will Start Where Others Stop. We can achieve any goal if we have that mindset. You can transform your fitness or change career; be a happier, kinder and more balanced person, parent and friend. Your community believes in you. I believe in you. Take a moment to really notice that feeling, to breathe it in and let it fill you up.

Because by getting started and setting a target towards something you are passionate about, committing to each stage of the process, celebrating your progress and using setbacks as launch pads, then building a team of like-minded people who support you as much as you now believe in yourself, you have done everything in your power to make it to your dream. When we get there, let's make sure we do a lot of dancing.

YOUR SWOS PROGRAMME

For this part of your Start Where Others Stop programme, you're going to reflect upon how far you've come. You've heard my story and how it shaped my mindset and you too have been on your own journey, from setting goals to overcoming hurdles and now how to achieve anything. Whether you've completed all or some of the exercises and reflections along the way or just found food for thought so far, all your progress is valuable and worthy of celebration.

So, at this point, we're going to look back over some of the major milestones we've covered in this book. Under each of the following headings, I'm going to ask you to list three things in your notebook or on the template on page 240. There are no examples here: this is a clean slate for you to fill with your own notes. If you have more to say, write down as many things as you like. If you have fewer, that's fine too. As we have learned, it's different for everyone and the process and practice is always the only aim.

1) WHAT THREE THINGS HAVE YOU ACHIEVED?

2) WHAT ARE YOUR THREE GREATEST STRENGTHS?

3) WHICH THREE ADVERSITIES HAVE YOU OVERCOME?

4) WHO ARE THREE PEOPLE WHO YOU HAVE SUPPORTED?

5) WHO ARE THREE PEOPLE WHO HAVE SUPPORTED YOU?

How did that make you feel? Wherever you are on your journey, you will have made some positive progress and this final evaluation should provide a shot of extra self-belief that you have taken steps to achieve, discovered your strengths and fostered a sense of teamwork and community. Even just picking up this book and reading this far is proof that you believe in your ability to become better.

CHAPTER NINE

GET READY TO START AGAIN

If you've followed the advice in this book, you will be well armed to attack your goals with a resilient mindset, focusing on the little wins and seeing the potential for growth through any setbacks. Maybe you've already made your first steps on your journey, resolving to make a start, planning out the smaller steps you need to take along the way, safe in the knowledge that, although your desired end point may change in time, you've looked back to understand the value of how far you've already come. Through the exercises in the SWOS programme at the end of each chapter, you have started to construct your own, personalised method of thinking, planning and progressing towards your unique goals.

When you get to your destination, you should take some time to enjoy yourself but you can't stop for too long. Because, the truth is, that fully embodying the Start Where Others Stop mindset means starting again. Reaching your goal, or changing it due to circumstances out of your direct control, is simply an opportunity to take stock and reset, to establish new objectives based on everything you have learned.

Even for CrossFit's ultra-elite, there are always countless areas in which to improve. You can always get fitter and become stronger or find a way to move better and with more skill. The best athletes in any sport, the smartest minds in business and the happiest people at home are so successful because they are constantly setting themselves new goals. They achieve, evaluate, set new goals and then start again. Tiger Woods didn't stop constantly refining his golf game when he won his first Major, after all.

Transformation of any sort is not a linear process and on the path from A to Z you have to pass the other 24 letters. There is no other way. If your dream is a big one, you will need to evaluate, adapt and start again as you move through the process.

On a fundamental level, to Start Where Others Stop you need to ensure you're always moving forwards. Starting again simply means you have a new expanse of open road in front of you. Let's all keep running.

CrossFit, as a sport, is all about starting again. Getting to the Regionals level in 2018 was a big milestone and one I genuinely enjoyed but missing out on qualifying for the CrossFit Games in 2019 was not part of the plan. After that, I had to draw a line and begin again almost immediately. That Open came in two parts for me, split down the middle by strict handstand push-ups: the first section when I was at the top of the leader board and was confident I could win, the second was finishing the last two workouts to the best of my ability, despite the disappointment. I changed my mindset and started again with a new short-term goal – to perform to the best of my abilities in the rest of the events.

It meant I came away from that competitive season in a positive mental space, rather than having to repair my confidence over the coming months, and hitting reset within the process kept me focused and happy. The plan was to win and become the UK national champion but I had to adapt in order to stay on course, so I started again by building to qualify through a Sanctional. When all the Sanctional events were finished and I still hadn't punched my ticket to Madison, I was officially not going to CrossFit Games. In 2019 I genuinely thought I'd make it and achieve my overarching goal.

So we evaluated the season by looking at the past year of training, competing and everything else that goes into being a professional athlete. I worked out what went right and what went wrong. Then we started again for the next season with a really solid plan in place, addressing my weaknesses to ensure I don't make the same mistakes again.

EVALUATION IN REAL LIFE

Self-assessment might sound like a chore but in reality evaluating your own behaviour is a process that can be extremely helpful to any part of your life.

If you always struggle to sleep on Sunday nights, evaluate what you're doing right, like not looking at your phone in bed or cutting out caffeine after midday. Consider what you could do better, such as staying consistent with your bed time even at the weekend or writing Monday's to-do list on a Sunday afternoon.

All you need to do is make a plan to address one, some or all of those factors, then start again next week. If you get to sleep quicker having adapted your routine, evaluate again what you did differently to identify the positively impactful changes. With a bit of self-assessment, improvement becomes an inevitability.

The Open in 2020 obviously went a lot better and winning was an achievement I'd been working towards with every workout and every handstand push-up since the previous year. Even within that successful five weeks, though, I was starting again almost constantly, repeating workouts with different tactics over and over, either to just try to go quicker or to find a strategy to get around my physique or injury-prone lower body.

That proved to me that even if everything goes to plan and you achieve your goal, there's still so much deviation, so much change that needs to take place in order to get there. I was the UK's fittest man and I had really grafted for it. But with that goal achieved and celebrated, I had to start again to begin prepping for the CrossFit Games. I had to move into a new training block and bring in all the unique movements and disciplines that you see at the next level – heavier weights, swimming, running, odd-object work and longer duration workouts.

When Coronavirus swept the world and everything changed, I again had to start from scratch. I was now getting ready for the 2021 season with a new plan in place to make it my strongest year ever. There are so many different points throughout a normal CrossFit season, let alone the strange nature of last year, where you start and start again. You're constantly changing strategies, learning from your mistakes, dealing with things that are totally out of your control and adapting to them. Again and again, you start a new plan and a new training programme. That's just part of sport.

Take something as singular as improving your bench press. If you hit a new personal best weight, you can't just go heavier next time. You need to work out what to change and what needs to improve to increase the weight. Is it your basic strength, or the minutiae of technique that goes into each lift? What could you tweak in your training to strengthen each of the various parts of the overall movement? That planning process becomes increasingly important the higher you climb in any sport, as a few extra kilos, a bit more speed and slightly better skills become the difference between victory and defeat.

You can constantly re-evaluate and start again, making those little tweaks and making sure you're going in the right direction. I think about how I'm approaching different movements, checking in with myself to consider if my programme is covering all the bases. You've got to make sure you're not so proud in your plan that you're unprepared to change it.

Take pistol squats. As we know, I can't do too many pistol squats or my knee blows up. I can manage them when it comes to competitions but in training, I need to go back to basics and be sensible. I do pistol squats with one foot on a box, so I can keep my foot flat and not put too much pressure through my ankle and knee. It's one of the ways we make it easier for new members but it works for me, an elite athlete, to go back to the beginning. I'm still working my glutes and hamstrings and quads and still getting through that movement, whereas if I was just to bang out loads of pistols, I know it would put me out of training and I would feel it in my ankles for a couple of weeks after.

There are a lot of things that I need to adjust for myself.

As a bigger athlete, I'm naturally strong, so I don't spend a lot of time doing out-and-out strength work. I do a few sessions here and there but I've never been on a strength cycle in the gym because I know that's going to be a waste of valuable time. If I don't practise my gymnastics regularly, however, it really shows. If I neglect it in my programme for a month, or after taking some time off from training, it just disappears. It's simple numbers: the total of reps I can do of pull-ups, say, is lower than it was before. At 100kg, it's not easy for me to jump onto a bar and start working through big sets, so I need to stay much more consistent with all of those movements in order that they don't limit my performance in competitions. You have to do your best to understand what parts of your life you are naturally capable in and which need more regular attention.

IMAGINE YOUR NEXT STEP

A gradual loss of motivation while moving towards a long-term goal is a natural inevitability, thanks to a psychological tendency called 'reward delay', which decreases our ability to value benefits that are going to occur in the future. It is a result of our evolutionary habit of preferring immediate gratification over long-term benefits, as our ancestors were more likely to survive if they used their resources immediately, rather than saving them for an unknown future. But neuroscientists at the University of Hamburg have found that you can work around our evolutionary tendencies with the power of 'episodic future thinking' – imagining yourself in future experiences in as much detail as possible.

If you relate episodic future thinking to your goals, you have a neurological way to combat reward delay. When forming a new goal, consider how reaching your goal would make you feel, how it would look, when you would like to achieve it and who else it would positively impact. Then simply repeat whenever you need to boost your motivation.

Self-evaluation is an incredible tool for ensuring you're always moving forwards. I think a lot of people get very carried away with hitting a goal and then just being happy with that and then that's that. My mentality is to achieve what I set out to do, then start the next journey. You celebrate what you've done and you evaluate what's worked well and not so well, decide what needs to change to make your progress even more successful. What can you do now to make things even better? Then you can set your sights on a new objective or reach for a higher level.

It means that if you reach a barrier, one that you can't just work harder in order to get over, you can start again with a positive mindset, focusing on the value of your experience and the growth that can come out of it. Closing the commercial gym and opening CrossFit BFG separated only by a handful of weeks and a few hundred yards is a clear example of this. So many people would have stopped but I was ready and willing to give it a go, understand where I could improve and then get onto it. It's an incredible feeling to pick yourself up when most would not expect you to, to dust yourself off and then set off straight away with a new plan and the same energy and excitement. And the more you do it, the better it gets. You become a person who does not settle, never stops and always aims high. You will become a person with a Start Where Others Stop mindset.

I always ask myself what I can achieve next. Let's say I get to the CrossFit Games in 2021, crush every workout and finish in the top ten. I would have hit every goal I have set for myself for the season and I could finally cross out the goal that has been on my board for all those years. But I would immediately start figuring out where to go from there. Perhaps I would decide to dial things back for a year and focus on my business career, or maybe Sam and I would start our own family. All goals are equal and you may choose to go in a different direction than before and that's perfect. As long as you're still moving, there is always more road to run.

Just before I started writing this book, I set a new personal best for handstand push-ups. I managed 31 reps without stopping. It was a huge win for me and, for my size, it was a

YOUR SWOS PROGRAMME

However you have transformed or improved, whether that is a physical change like mine as a child, or a mental shift as a result of a setback, such as missing the chance to qualify for the CrossFit Games when it was well within reach, it's fair to say we've all come a long way. Perhaps your own journey is just beginning or maybe you've achieved your dream and want to set your sights higher.

What will have developed in the course of reading this book and using the tools we've worked on together is your skill at goal setting, self-awareness and ability to honestly and openly appraise your performance.

For this last part of your Start Where Others Stop programme, you're going to reflect upon your goal-setting methodology, reviewing the stages of the plan you've been creating as we've moved through the chapters together. Take some time to look over all the notes you've made while reading this book and celebrate how far you've come or be excited about where you're going to go next. On the following page, there's a summary of the whole programme so if you missed any stage or feel like you didn't cover it properly, go back and give it a go.

PART I: SET GOALS

1) MAKE A START
First of all, contemplate setting a goal by considering both your background and your desired future. Ask yourself who you are, where you would like to go and what will get you there.

2) TAKE SMALL STEPS
Work on refining your goals and establishing the micro-goals that will be integral in measured and positive progress. Assess your goals to ensure they are precise, challenging and clear.

3) PURSUE YOUR PASSION
Evaluate your progress and ensure your goal is aligned with something you are truly passionate about by working how you would feel if you achieved your goal and how it would feel were you not to.

PART II: OVERCOME CHALLENGES

4) COMMIT TO THE MOMENT

Understand that enjoying yourself as much as you're able to is a way of topping up your fuel tank of motivation, then put that to the test by pledging to make small improvements towards an achievable milestone.

5) FIND STRENGTH IN WEAKNESS

Apply the same specificity to your perceived weakness as you do to your strengths. Take something you view as an inability, imagine how it could become a positive and then identify how to make that transformation.

6) USE SETBACKS AS LAUNCH PADS

Grasp how failure is a contributor to success and then understand setbacks are a chance to make a comeback by seeing the situation as a whole, separating yourself from an overly emotional response and focusing on what you can do tomorrow.

PART III: ACHIEVE ANYTHING

7) FIND YOUR COMMUNITY

Unlock the mutually rewarding benefits of community and support the other people around you when they need you, remembering to offer your help before being asked, listen without trying to relate it to your experience and treat each person and/or instance as unique.

8) FIND YOUR SELF-BELIEF

Look back at your progress and achievements to see the value in your actions and find the self-belief to make further improvement. List your strengths and success-es, the adversities you have overcome and people you have supported or been supported by.

9) GET READY TO START AGAIN

Review your SWOS programme and look back at your journey so far. If you've achieved your goal, can you aim higher with the new knowledge you've acquired? If your goal needs changing, you have the tools you need to start again and be more successful. Good luck!

YOUR SWOS PROGRAMME
EXERCISE TEMPLATES

Introduction

To help as a reminder for the exercises below, write down your goal here. This might change as you go through the SWOS programme and that's OK! This is just to get us started.

_____

_____

_____

PART I: SET GOALS

Chapter 1: Anyone Can Make a Start

Who are you?

Firstly, consider the three defining characteristics of your personality (both positive and negative).

1. _____
2. _____
3. _____

Now, write down who or what is responsible for instilling those traits. It might be family members, friends, the school you went to, and so on. Don't forget to think about how you've contributed to these too.

_____
_____
_____
_____
_____
_____
_____

Where would you like to go?

Look back at the goal you've written at the start of this section. Taking into account everything you've written above, do you feel like this is still the right destination for you? If you want to revise it, write your new goal here.

_____

_____

_____

_____

_____

_____

_____

What will get you there?

Finally, let's identify the primary positive action that will get you to your goal. What change can you make that will have the largest impact? Be ambitious but also truthful to what you think will be best for you.

_____

_____

_____

_____

_____

_____

_____

Chapter 2: Take Small Steps to Achieve Big Dreams

Be precise. Now that you've learned the importance of taking small steps, write down your goal again but this time, be as precise as possible – what is it that you *really* want to achieve?

_____

_____

_____

_____

_____

_____

_____

Now have a think about exactly how you're going to measure your success and track your milestones – what are the tangible ways you can note your progress?

_____

_____

_____

_____

_____

_____

_____

_____

Be challenged. Is your goal too easy for you? If you think 'No way, this is definitely a stretch', then great, leave it as is. If it's looking too simple, however, take a moment now to make it a bit harder. You want to be pushing yourself.

_____

_____

_____

_____

_____

_____

_____

_____

_____

_____

_____

_____

_____

_____

_____

Be clear. You will only achieve your goal if you break it down into smaller parts. Use the table on the opposite page to think about the mid- and short-term goals you can achieve that will eventually help you get to your main goal.

	Mid-term goals (what can you achieve in a month?)	Short-term goals (what can you achieve in a week or day?)
My main goal is to . . .		

Chapter 3: Pursue Your Passion

It's time to focus on how you *feel*. This can't be underestimated and being honest to yourself about how you're feeling is key to achieving your goal. This might be a little uncomfortable to begin with, so if you need to come back to this after a shower, or even a week after mulling it over, that's fine.

How will I feel when I achieve my goal?	How will I feel if I don't achieve my goal?

PART II: OVERCOME CHALLENGES

Chapter 4: Commit to the Moment

Choose one of your short-term goals from p. 231 that you can track here. How are you going to build on this goal? Will you increase the intensity of the action, or maybe do it more frequently? Write down your intention here and then set a reminder on your phone for this time next week.

Also, make a note of how you will celebrate achieving your goal! Perhaps it will be sharing the news with a loved one or posting something on your socials. Maybe it'll be giving yourself time for a bath or making time for that TV show you've always wanted to watch. Big or small, write it down.

My intention is to. . .

_____

_____

_____

_____

_____

_____

_____

I will celebrate by . . .

_____

_____

_____

_____

_____

_____

_____

_____

_____

_____

_____

_____

Chapter 5: Find Strength in Weakness

This is perhaps one of the most challenging aspects of working towards anything – failure. We've all been there and the most useful tool I've learned is to be as specific about my *inabilities* as I am about my abilities. Not only does this ensure I'm not exaggerating what I can't do, but it helps me recognise what I can do – it's a win, win!

Fill in the table on the opposite page and use the examples on p. 142 if you're struggling to get started.

YOUR SWOS PROGRAMME EXERCISE TEMPLATES

Weaknesses	Strengths	Changes

Chapter 6: Use Setbacks as Launchpads

Consider all the angles. You're ready to make your comeback and you'll do this by firstly recognising other forces that might have affected your performance. This might be an unrelated personal event that happened the day before and threw you off your game, perhaps the weather was appalling, maybe your partner was going through something and that required most of your focus. Take some time to write down the external factors here:

_____

_____

_____

_____

_____

_____

_____

_____

_____

Be a 'situation' solver. While it's always important to recognise how you're feeling, you also want to separate your emotions from a situation to see them most clearly. We're going to consider what steps you can make to improve and move forward. On the following page, as before, make a note in the table of your mid- and short-term goals.

	Mid-term goals (what can you achieve in a month?)	Short-term goals (what can you achieve in a week or day?)
I've experienced a setback however I'm ready for my comeback. My new goal is to . . .		

And finally, **focus on tomorrow.** Circle or underline the goal in the right column that you will do tomorrow. I know you can do it.

PART III: ACHIEVE ANYTHING

Chapter 7: Find Your Community

Don't make them ask for help. I couldn't be where I am today without the love and support of those around me. But we need to give, as much as we receive, to fully unlock the rewarding benefits of community. Write down someone you can help (even if they haven't asked for your help) and a specific, tangible way you can help them.

_____

_____

_____

Don't make it about you. Being a good listener is hard! It takes practice and it doesn't always come naturally to people. If you're someone who, with good intentions, always ends up relating people's experiences back to your own, have a think about ways you can respond that keep the focus on the other person. For example:

That sounds _____ is there anything I can do to help?
I can understand why that must feel _____.

What are you going to do next?

Make a note of any other responses that come to mind, so you can be the best possible support for your friend, family member or colleague in need next time.

_____

_____

_____

_____

_____

_____

_____

_____

_____

_____

_____

_____

Don't forget the person. This is just something to remember. Everyone is different and so everyone needs a unique form of support. When the people in a community all support one another, it gives every person the belief that they can be their full selves. By properly helping others, you're in turn also helping yourself.

Chapter 8: Build Your Self-Belief

It's time to reflect. Answer the questions below, if you can't think of three for each, that's OK.

What three things have you achieved?

1. _____
2. _____
3. _____

What are your three greatest strengths?

1. _____
2. _____
3. _____

Which three adversities have you overcome?

1. _____
2. _____
3. _____

Who are three people you have supported?

1. _____
2. _____
3. _____

Who are three people who have supported *you*?

1. _____
2. _____
3. _____

Take a moment to reflect on how answering those questions made you feel.

_____
_____
_____
_____
_____
_____
_____
_____

Chapter 9: Get Ready to Start Again

Well done! You've come to the end of your SWOS Pro-gramme. Go back over the answers you've recorded on these pages and consider what worked for you and what didn't. If you've still got work to do on achieving your goal – go for it! You've got this. If you're ready for a new goal though, copy out the questions and tables above and go again. I believe in you.

ACKNOWLEDGEMENTS

First, I would like to thank my mum and my dad. My parents are my idols; they have shown me what is possible with hard work and have always taught me to aim high. They have given me the mentality I have today which I am so grateful for.

My sister, Martine, has also always been there for me and supported me in absolutely anything I have done in life. She is my number one fan and the person who is screaming the loudest in my corner.

To James Sealey, my manager and good friend, I'm lucky to have someone who is so professional and good at their job but who I also get on *so* well with. James allows me to focus on my training, takes away a lot of the stress and handles all of my sponsorships and brand activity. James is a person I look up to and I'm so fortunate to have in my corner.

My business partner and good friend Harmeet Singh is the person who first taught me CrossFit and who believed that one day I could qualify for the CrossFit Games. Seven years later, we achieved that goal and he has been there right beside me the whole way.

Ben Bodycombe doesn't programme for me as I do that myself, but he always has the coaches pass at all my competitions. He plays a massive role in me competing at my best, and handles absolutely everything for me during competitions, from my food to warm-up times and workout strategies. I can rely on him 100 per cent to help with anything I need and that is something I will never take for granted.

Daniel Wagner is my training partner and a good friend. Dan plays a huge part in keeping me motivated and making sure my training is fun and enjoyable. We train together every single day and he is always there when I need a pick-up of motivation and he keeps me in line. The world's best CrossFit domestique.

Vivek Saundh is my best friend, he doesn't have much to do with my current career but I've known him for 15-plus years and I don't think there have been many days where we haven't spoken on the phone. He is the person who no matter what was going on, whatever the issue or subject, he would be the first one I'd call.

John Chapman is another best friend who I look up to greatly and who, along with Leon Bustin, showed me the possibilities of social media. Both of them are always at competitions to support me no matter where in the world it's taking place and John is often the one I'll look to for advice on anything in terms of career and training. There have been many times during workouts in competitions where I've looked for John in the crowd seeking his valuable advice.

Josh Burniston is another training partner, close friend and someone I've watched grow from a shy young lad into one of the head coaches at my gym, CrossFit BFG. Josh and Harmeet take so much off my plate and allow me to focus heavily on training whilst they look after all the complex day-to-day running and maintenance of the box.

Finally, every successful man has a strong woman behind them. Samantha Brown is that strong woman for me. She is always there with me during all my ups and downs and will always be the person I most rely upon, every single day.

Zack George is one of the world's top athletes and officially the UK's fittest man.

Known within the CrossFit® community as 'Silverback', Zack is one of the most influential figures in the sport. He is the founder of Silverback Training, a fitness influencer with over 190K followers, and was named one of '13 Inspirational Black Men Who Are Leading their Fields and Paving the Way for the Next Generation' by Men's Health Online. He has been the cover star for *Men's Health* Magazine and has been featured in British *GQ*, *MAN Magazine*, *Men's Fitness*, The Sportsman, Business Insider, Man of Many, JOE.co.uk, Yahoo and more.

Zack lives in Leicester, UK with his girlfriend Sam and their puppy Layla. This is his first book.